THE
HELPERS

THE
HELPERS

Profiles from the Front Lines
of the Pandemic

KATHY GILSINAN

W. W. NORTON & COMPANY
Independent Publishers Since 1923

A. W. "Smokey" Linn, "Fireman's Prayer," 1958. Reprinted with permission of
Penny McGlachlin.

For information about permission to reproduce selections from this book, write to
Permissions, W. W. Norton & Company, Inc., 500 Fifth Avenue,
New York, NY 10110

For information about special discounts for bulk purchases, please contact
W. W. Norton Special Sales at specialsales@wwnorton.com or 800-233-4830

Manufacturing by Lakeside Book Company
Book design by Ellen Cipriano
Production manager: Lauren Abbate

ISBN 978-0-393-86702-2

W. W. Norton & Company, Inc., 500 Fifth Avenue, New York, N.Y. 10110
www.wwnorton.com

W. W. Norton & Company Ltd., 15 Carlisle Street, London W1D 3BS

1 2 3 4 5 6 7 8 9 0

For Mom and Dad
Selfless helpers, dear friends, and north star(s) to your girl
Thank you.

All the darkness in the world cannot extinguish the light of a single candle.

—SAINT FRANCIS OF ASSISI

. . . To state plainly what we learn in times of pestilence: that there are more things to admire in men than to despise.

—ALBERT CAMUS, *THE PLAGUE*

We can only do what we can: but that we must do, against difficulties.

—ISAIAH BERLIN, "THE PURSUIT OF THE IDEAL"

CONTENTS

PART THREE

A NOTE ON THE SOURCES

THIS BOOK TELLS the story of America's Covid pandemic through the accounts of people with a direct role in fighting it. In all but one case, the protagonists themselves told me their stories over multiple conversations through 2020 and early 2021; where the book "gets into their heads," describing their feelings or thoughts, the material comes from their own recollections to me. Dialogue is generally rendered as the book's main characters recalled it in our interviews. In the case where the protagonist is deceased, I have reconstructed his story through interviews with family members and colleagues who witnessed his activities in his early career and during the Covid crisis, or spoke to him during the events described—descriptions of his thoughts and feelings are secondhand, from people who told me what he told them, or taken from his own Facebook posts.

Readers should view Covid-related statistics cited here as best available contemporaneous estimates, bearing in mind that, especially in early 2020, the counts are imprecise. Testing shortages in the United States early in 2020 prevented a full accounting of the virus's spread, but even with testing improvements, serious data problems persisted—the quality of the data varies with the state health department collecting it. The numbers should be read as a rough sense of the pandemic's scale as officials saw it on any given day.

Finally, the individuals quoted here do not represent the institutions for which they work. Michelle Gonzalez, for example, speaks for herself, and not for Montefiore Health System or the Moses campus where she serves.

INTRODUCTION

T HE PANDEMIC HAPPENED to us one by one. We were isolated, we were trapped with family; we got tired of remote work, we tried to earn money while educating homebound children, we got laid off, we risked health to show up to jobs that were somehow both "essential" and poorly compensated; we escaped infection, we got sick, we had no symptoms or mild symptoms or severe symptoms, we went on ventilators, we recovered, we lost loved ones or friends of friends, we died by the hundreds of thousands.

In the United States, the catastrophe seemed slow until it was sudden, and remote until it was everywhere. We ignored it in late 2019 and early 2020 or watched it gather—first with a few disquieting headlines about a new illness in China, a smattering of warnings about what could happen here. We feared those warnings or didn't notice them or dismissed them as alarmist—after all, influenza killed tens of thousands of people a year in the United States, and how bad could this be?

The virus leapt out of Asia. Cases exploded in Iran and then Italy, where doctors were forced to ration care and leave some of the most vulnerable to die. A few drips and then a flood of infections developed in the United States, but most of us didn't understand exponential growth, that a mere 15 confirmed instances in mid-February would mean 1,000 in less than a month; that in the beginning it would take at least three months to detect a million new coronavirus disease (Covid) cases, and by November only 10 days. California shut down in mid-March. A cascade of states followed. By the end of March, the United States was the pandemic's global epicenter.

We were not prepared. The president had told us in January that the virus in the United States, then consisting of a single reported case, was totally under control; he then warned in March that the country could see up to a quarter of a million deaths from the disease it caused. By Christmastime it was clear that even that formerly unthinkable figure had been an underestimate, and America closed out 2020 with more than 340,000 of its people dead from a scourge we'd barely heard of when the year started. By the following summer, the American toll had climbed past 600,000.

But in the early days, when we saw how drastically life had to change but didn't yet understand the scale and duration of the disaster bearing down on us, we could fairly easily locate hope. In March and April of 2020 we saw the first round of the worst of it, but also glimmers of the best of us. We went grocery shopping for homebound neighbors or stuck teddy bears in our windows for kids to spot on walks around the neighborhood; we sewed masks in our homes or businesses; we converted booze distilleries into hand-sanitizer factories; we found ways to make one another less lonely. We launched pen-pal programs with nursing homes and "Quarantine Buddy" software to randomly match people in video chats now that serendipitous encounters—or, for some of us, any encounters—were rare. Human invention met human compassion, over and over.

Even the 116th Congress, one of the least productive in decades and fresh off a bitter impeachment fight, managed to come together that first pandemic March to send help, offering an economic lifeline to struggling businesses and citizens to the tune of more than $2 trillion, with other measures to support paid sick leave, unemployment benefits, and vaccine research. Most Americans seemed to believe, and behave as if, we were all in this together. Nothing underscores human interconnectedness quite like contagion, and if one person could, through absentmindedness, denial, or malice, cause a cascade of disease and death for those with the misfortune to cross his path, so much more did this reinforce the central truth: We had to take care of each other.

We did this by the millions, staying home or keeping our distance, wearing masks to stop the spread of infection. We upended our routines and deprived ourselves of the comfort of family and friends even as we lived through crisis and longed for reassurance. We endured a national trauma orders of magnitude deadlier than the 9/11 attacks, and though people around the country overwhelmed blood banks with donations in response to that horror, 9/11 brought with it no long-standing nationwide effort to help and to protect one another. The biggest burdens then were borne by the few—police officers, firefighters, EMTs, and other first responders, including local volunteers who rushed to the scene in New York and in Washington, and then, in the wars that followed the attacks, the members of the military, many of whom would go on to multiple deployments over the next 20 years. But these were a small proportion of the overall population. Most Americans could indulge, if they wanted to, in the luxury of tuning out the wars. Our then-president encouraged us not to be scared away from shopping, to get down to Disney World, to enjoy our lives.

As much as that may have been a defiant response to a terrorist threat, it wasn't a national call to communal caring. Seven years later, the country suffered a different kind of historically destructive shock in the 2008 global financial crisis, whose costs Americans shouldered all over the country; taxpayers bailed out banks while millions of people lost jobs, savings, and homes. In rescuing the financial system we may have saved each other from much worse economic pain, but if this was a form of societal solidarity, most of us had no individual say in it.

The scale of collective mobilization Americans displayed in the spring of 2020 was more reminiscent of the home-front solidarity of World War II. Then, private citizens across the country conducted scrap-metal and rubber drives to keep the troops supplied from their own possessions; children tended victory gardens to supplement rations and feed their neighborhoods. The war bonds that people purchased helped finance the fighting, but then-president Franklin Delano Roosevelt also promoted them as a way to foster a collective sense of purpose, of being in it together.

Our version of mass action looked decidedly passive in comparison—one meme that circulated in the spring admonished: "Your grandparents were called to war. You're being called to sit on your couch. You can do this." This was early, before anyone yet understood the depth of sacrifice such a call would entail, and the enormous economic and social costs that isolation and shutdown would exact—10 million net jobs lost by the end of the year, tens of thousands of bankruptcies, entire people-facing industries such as restaurants devastated, record drug overdose deaths. Americans were in fact being called to endure historic hardships, on top of the millions who would be infected and the hundreds of thousands who would die.

The results, as anyone should expect from such a catalog of horrors, included rancor and division, political ineptitude and buck-passing, fury at leaders and fellow citizens for restricting too much or not enough or insisting on masks or refusing to wear them. Almost as soon as there were shortages, there were counterfeits and price gouging. As soon as there were mask mandates, there was violence over them.

But the results of pandemic hardship also, less expectedly and more importantly, included an outburst of altruism that saved lives and fed the hungry. Social-distancing guidelines across the country, even the most onerous state stay-at-home orders, relied for the most part on voluntary compliance, and for the most part, according to national polls taken in 2020, people did comply. The majority of the country did this despite the missteps, confusion, denial, and buck-passing of the federal response, in which the president left states and localities to formulate wildly differing containment measures and scramble for tests and protective equipment, contributing to hundreds of thousands of deaths that could have been stopped. This wasn't China, where health officials went door-to-door to hunt down and isolate the sick; nor even France, where people had to carry forms with them attesting to their approved reason for leaving the house. While news reports displayed images of packed bars in states with looser virus-mitigation measures and of anti-mask protesters hoisting signs about tyranny in stricter states, the truth was that most Americans reported practicing social distancing and wearing masks to leave the house, making millions of difficult, boring, unglamorous decisions to protect their neighbors, adding up to an act of mass kindness. These acts weren't newsworthy precisely because they were the norm for ordinary citizens; denial and callousness were not.

In fact, a major reason social distancing was such a hardship for us is that human beings love other human beings. Meanwhile, the disease was showing us both how our fates depended on one another's behavior and how easily our fellow man's suffering could become our own. It was easy to feel compassion for the sick, the suffering, the out of work, because we all to one degree or another faced many of the same risks. We all lost something. This is not to say the effects were felt equally—the sick, the poor, the elderly, and communities of color bore by far the worst of them—but everybody felt them.

It was easy, too, to feel gratitude for those whose ordinary jobs now put them on the "front lines" of a war for which nobody had volunteered. The country elevated a new class of heroes: not the celebrities and other assorted high rollers who normally reaped praise and credit in this country, but the people who had been there all along, helping keep everyone safe and fed, who were now shouldering deadly risks to do so. No less elitist a publication than the *Financial Times*, home of a "luxury lifestyle" magazine supplement for the ultra-rich called *How to Spend It*, ran a story calling truckers "heroes of the highway"; giant corporations including Walmart were suddenly at pains to run tender commercials praising workers.

There will be other books written on the many ways we failed these individuals and each other, about the bungled government response, about how the arc of American public life bent from goodwill toward dysfunction. There will be eloquent condemnations of Washington politicians who spent an election year collecting six-figure salaries and soliciting campaign donations while failing for eight months to extend more support to the needy—and then cut many first responders in line for vaccines. Other authors will investigate the corporations that hailed their hero workers as a public-relations strategy but refused to protect them with adequate equipment or to offer better wages and paid sick leave. The leadership blunders of this era will serve as a warning to future generations.

The Helpers tells a parallel yet no less true story of the pandemic in the United States, because the truth is that most people behaved honorably, and the fact that they did so in spite of harrowing circumstances and bad leadership makes their efforts even more worthy of celebration.

So this is a book about ordinary people who stepped up to meet an extraordinary moment and persisted in determination to help others, even as the temptation of hopelessness lurked. They don't have much in common; they come from all over the country, and most have never met. But they all embody the best of America while the worst rages around them. They include a well-beloved and mustachioed paramedic from Denver who drives an ambulance across the country, despite age and doubtful health, straight into the peak of New York's surge. A brassy Bronx nurse who witnesses the trauma of an overwhelmed hospital and the infection of her own parents. A slick young CEO running a small ventilator company outside Seattle who forges an impossible partnership with an auto manufacturer in a scramble to prevent shortages. An unassuming program leader at an unproven Boston biotech firm who persuades skeptical bosses to stake everything on a race for the vaccine. A determined twenty-something teacher and chef in Louisville who launches a community kitchen to feed the hungry in a wounded community longing for racial justice. Threaded through their stories is that of a Covid patient who battles the worst of the disease that drives the fates of the others in these pages, and whose ordeal shows the face of the enemy we're all up against.

None of them necessarily had an extraordinary sense of faith that they could make things all right or even be all right themselves. What they did have was an extraordinary sense of stubbornness. It's easy enough to have faith when things are getting better. It seems so quaint now to think how, early in this disease's progress in the United States, many of us thought that a few weeks of partial hunkering down would be enough to save us. The president promulgated modest plans, suggesting on March 16, 2020, that Americans take steps, such as staying home when sick and keeping away from others if suffering from serious underlying health conditions, for "15 Days to Slow the Spread." But weeks unspooled into months, and the end date to the life disruptions kept receding or disappeared altogether as death hit our families and changed our worlds forever. We, and the people in these pages, watched horizons of hope disappear one by one—first summer, when we were told perhaps the heat could kill the virus, but instead we watched it catch fire in new regions of the country; then the holiday season, when many of us faced the wrenching choice between being with loved ones after such long loneliness and dread or playing it safe as the experts warned of a horrifying flood of cases and pleaded with us to stay home. In each case the moment of hope gave way to a period of renewed fear. We were punished for our yearnings for togetherness with yet more infections.

The true test of faith is whether you can retain it when things are getting worse. But the test of a whole person is whether you can keep showing up when you've lost faith entirely. Good deeds needed to get done, no matter the belief that they were leading toward anything sustainably better.

All of the people described in these pages faced extreme doubts, the knowledge that they couldn't save everyone, and the risk of falling ill themselves. They were all up against a force of nature, the enormity of which could feel helpless-making, flaunting as it did the smallness of human strivings like the ocean to a lonely sunbather. That the force took the form of an invisible nanoparticle, wantonly smashing human lives and human plans, was a crueler mockery of our illusions about our own power. Yet it ultimately fell to humans to defeat it. And so these remarkable people, and many others like them, kept showing up anyway.

There's a scene in *The Plague*, Albert Camus's classic novel of a fictional pestilence in 1940s Oran, Algeria, in which "fledgling moralists" advise that nothing can be done and the townspeople might as well give up. Dr. Rieux and his companions can only offer "their certitude that a fight must be put up, in this way or that, and there must be no bowing down."

So many of our own plague's fighters, including the people

in this book, would likely recognize Dr. Rieux's quotidian struggles. "There's no question of heroism in all this," the doctor at one point tells his friend. "It's a matter of common decency. That's an idea which may make some people smile, but the only means of fighting a plague is—common decency." Whatever that means for other people, he says, "In my case I know that it consists in doing my job."

Now more than 700,000 lives have been lost, and the fight is not yet finished. Though scientists have developed multiple vaccines in record time, lighting our way to the end of the scourge, it's difficult to predict the remaining course of the disease in America, much less what Americans will rebuild from the wreckage. Past periods of economic contortion and deprivation such as occurred during World War II saw American society reshaped over decades, as the mobilization of women into factory work, and the sacrifices of African Americans on behalf of a country that still treated them as second-class citizens, respectively laid the groundwork for the women's liberation and civil rights movements. A better post-pandemic world is possible, but it isn't inevitable. What we do with the pandemic's lessons—about the weaknesses of our public-health system, the gaps in our social safety net, deadly racial inequality, and the meaning of "essential" work—is in our hands.

I hope we are laying the groundwork for a better society we can't yet clearly see, precisely because this pandemic has exposed the ways our society is broken now. This is the story of how we beat the pandemic, but I hope that it someday serves as an introduction to the story of how we made a better country.

That future starts with people like the ones in this book.

PART ONE

The Patient

Sick

Huy Le wrenched himself out of bed at an awful predawn hour because that's what a good little brother does. His sister Uyên's flight to Chicago for a teaching seminar was departing around 5:00 a.m. on March 16, and naturally it was his job to ferry her through the dark quiet to the San Jose airport from their parents' house just north of the city. Huy took the responsibility; everyone else could sleep.

Uyên planned to leave her two-year-old son, Kai, with her parents while she traveled, then retrieve him on her way back home to her husband and her job as a family medicine doctor in Nevada. Creeping out of the house that spring morning, Huy found his mom dozing on the couch and asked her softly to go check on the little one and sleep in his room in case he woke up needing something. His mom muttered a foggy assent. "Okay, go."

Huy had his own place, a condo in San Francisco, financed by long employment with Silicon Valley tech giants—10 years at Apple and another 7 months at Facebook. But he still made a point to spend a night or two a week at his parents' place in Milpitas, the South Bay town where he grew up. This was only partly because doing so shaved off a lot of the commute time to the Facebook offices in Menlo Park. Mostly, he was close to his family, just as serious about being a son as being a little brother.

The Les were not "I love you" people, and when Huy was growing up his parents were more inclined to guilt him with tales of their immigrant struggles than comfort him for his own American-kid problems, which seemed pitifully small to them. They'd fled Vietnam on boats in the 1970s, worked their asses off to give their children a good California life, and the kid didn't like doing homework? He could get the heck over it. And incidentally should really be getting better grades.

They weren't much for hugging, either. They showed affection through time spent together and helping each other. Huy's mom cooked Vietnamese specialties for him when he came back—his favorite was a beef noodle soup from his dad's home region in Huế that, while available in Vietnamese restaurants, never turned out quite the same as it did at home. His parents always kept the fridge stocked for him. His sister came back for a long weekend about once a month.

All of this meant the old house in Milpitas maintained its appeal for Huy, property-owning mid-thirties bachelor that he was, even though, by that barely-even morning in March, the commute was no longer a factor. More than a week earlier, on March 5, Facebook had asked its workers to work remotely to keep from spreading the new coronavirus that had already been multiplying in the United

States for weeks. In those early days the novelty of not commuting, and being able to "show up" to video meetings in shorts, hadn't yet worn off. Huy was happy to avoid pants for as long as he could.

Meanwhile, his mom, a real-estate agent and devout Buddhist, had only stopped going to temple at her kids' insistence, just in case. Huy didn't even know if she was still showing properties, and she was still getting invited to housewarming parties for her clients—she'd taken his dad to one only the week before. The virus seemed very far away and theoretical, just numbers in newspapers, and small ones at that, though a few of the people behind them were disconcertingly close to Milpitas. In February, officials had disclosed two infections in the surrounding Santa Clara County. Both of those stricken with the illness the virus caused, formally dubbed COVID-19 for *coronavirus disease 2019*, had returned from Wuhan, China, where the new virus had first been detected.

By March 7 officials had identified 32 cases in the county, the most in the San Francisco Bay Area, and San Francisco's director of health was warning that the spread was accelerating. And the virus was showing up among people with absolutely no connection to Wuhan. One of them, a 68-year-old Iranian emigré named Azar Ahrabi, died on March 9. Santa Clara health officials believed at the time that Ahrabi, a genial mom who was caring for her own octogenarian mother and liked to befriend people at the grocery store, was the first person to have died of Covid in the Bay Area. Because she'd had no recent travel history, doctors who saw her at first dismissed the possibility she could be carrying the new virus. The day she died, a cruise ship with 21 known infections—as determined by tests helicoptered aboard and then helicoptered back to a lab while the ship circled off the coast of

San Francisco—docked in Oakland, and its thousands of passengers
were swept away to quarantine on military bases.

No one knew until weeks later that the virus had been circulating undetected far beyond the modest tallies being put out by
the Centers for Disease Control and Prevention (CDC), that in
fact it had been killing people in the Bay Area even before Ahrabi
died. Postmortem tests later showed that the virus had killed Patri-
cia Dowd, 57, in San Jose on February 6, making hers retroactively
the first known Covid death in the entire country. She hadn't traveled abroad for months prior to when her daughter reportedly found
her lying on the floor by her breakfast table. No one had tested her
for the virus when she exhibited flulike symptoms in February; the
CDC guidance at the time was to conserve scarce tests for returning overseas travelers. Another Californian was later found to have
died with the virus on February 17, and another on March 6. This
hidden death toll also obscured a much larger rate of infection,
weeks before the state would take any action to keep it in check.

The Le family had none of this information as Huy and Uyên
headed to San Jose; they knew what Covid was but didn't think it
particularly serious. Even Uyên, the doctor in the family, was non-
chalant. She had joked in the days prior to that car ride that she
wished she could just get the illness and get it over with. And then
she was on her way to schmooze with other medical professionals
in another city.

It was just about 6:00 a.m. when Huy came back to the house
and slipped into his nephew's room, expecting to see his mom there,
sleeping near the boy. But Kai was alone. Huy's mom was still lying
on the couch.

"Hey, is everything okay? Why aren't you with Kai?"

She told him she was feeling sick and didn't want to infect her grandson if it was something serious. That was Huy's first indication that everything was about to change.

■   ■   ■

Huy's mom and dad, Liên and Nghề, fell in love surrounded by the wreckage of war in Vietnam. Then, in 1978, when they were both in their early twenties, they fled the country.

The fall of Saigon to communist forces in 1975 only intensified the humanitarian disaster wrought by war. Communist rule brought widespread misery and deprivation; Nghề's father, for instance, had owned massive plots of farmland, which the government duly confiscated, leaving his family destitute. The young couple, not yet married, decided to take a gamble on a better life. They were part of a mass exodus of perhaps 800,000 so-called boat people who put themselves at the mercy of fickle seas and Thai pirates to escape, with unknown tens or hundreds of thousands dying in the attempt. The survivors faced other dangers, including prolonged detention in wretched regional refugee camps or being kidnapped and sold into slavery.

Liên left a few months before Nghề, on a large ship with roughly a hundred other people, all braving the four-day journey to Hong Kong. Nghề came later, on a much smaller boat, stuffed with more than a dozen people—sisters, children, friends. Nghề had to steer, and Huy heard many times growing up how his dad stayed awake for four days straight to guide the vessel over the South China Sea, sipping on a can of condensed milk to keep from dozing off.

Liên stayed in Hong Kong for only a few months and had already made it into the United States through a sponsorship program by the time Nghề arrived in Hong Kong. They wrote letters to one another as he worked to join her in America, but a snag in Nghề's U.S. visa paperwork kept him in Hong Kong for several additional months: Liên had marked herself single on her own application, but he had declared himself already married to her. A lawyer eventually sorted it out, and they reunited near San Jose and got married for real.

She got a job on the assembly line at Memorex to pay for his electrical engineering degree. Nghề picked up an American name, Nick, graduated, got a job of his own at a semiconductor company, Cirrus Logic, and started studying for an electrical engineering master's degree at night. Later, Liên and her sister-in-law opened a store, Campbell Liquors and Deli, on East Campbell Avenue in Campbell, California. The two kept the place open seven days a week, Liên taking one weekend day off and her sister the other. Nghề helped out at the store, too, in the few hours that his company or his studies didn't claim, coming straight to the store Friday nights after work, pitching in on weekends. Meanwhile, Liên devoted spare moments to community service, being active in her temple, helping sponsor others from Vietnam to start their lives in America, spotting opportunities to put a little more light into the world when she could.

Huy remembered childhood days in the back of the store—his parents couldn't really afford childcare—where he learned more than anybody his age should know about all kinds of liquor and how to distinguish the good vodka from the cheap stuff. As he got older, he and his sister helped out, scooping ice from the industrial ice maker in back into bags for the customers, restocking shelves, manning the register, assembling sandwiches. That was how Huy first developed his lifelong appreciation for a nice turkey–bacon–avocado combo and a taste for chips and corn nuts. Friday nights after school were busy as people stocked up on drinks for the weekend, and he and his sister might fill 20 or 30 bags of ice, a task Nghề would reward with an honorarium of 50 cents each. Huy might then ask for a snack from the shelf. "Sure," Nghề would say. "That will cost you 50 cents."

Huy and his sister later liked to joke that this was how they learned the value of money. Nothing in life came without work. Not a new start in America, not an engineering degree or a small business, not even corn nuts. Huy's parents had seen hell and risked death to build an American dream for their family, and now Huy was living in it. If that knowledge was a source of enormous pressure to make the most of it, to somehow earn retroactively what they had given him, it was also a filament in the bond that kept him close to his family, and an example for his own life. He walked his father's path and became an engineer.

■   ■   ■

The realm of West Coast tech where Huy ended up was among the first in America to dispatch armies of employees back to their own homes in retreat from the virus. The new, spikey little pathogen—measuring perhaps a thousandth the width of a human hair—became the puppeteer of multibillion-dollar companies much more accustomed to shaping the world themselves. Twitter, Amazon,

Microsoft, Google, and Facebook hollowed out their offices and tried to hide from infection. Self-described "tech bros" such as Huy parked their Teslas and forsook their pants.

It didn't occur to Huy that infection had arrived anyway, at home, slipping into his mom's lungs. That flu season had been especially vicious, so it seemed likely Liên's was a commonplace ailment, nothing the right mix of Gatorade, tea, and Tamiflu couldn't vanquish. His sister prescribed something, came back to retrieve her son after three days in Chicago, and headed home to Nevada, expecting her mom to get better soon.

But Liên's appetite continued to fade. She mostly just lay on the couch, aching, cramped, and feverish, while Huy urged her to eat. She refused nearly everything until Huy, in desperation, went straight at her sweet tooth with a cup of *chè*, her favorite Vietnamese dessert, made with red beans in a sugary syrup with coconut milk and jellies. Using the confection as a lure, he finally coaxed her off the couch and into the kitchen, where she trudged over to him, ate half, then returned to the couch, worn out from the trip.

On the morning of Thursday, March 19, Liên reported to her son that she was having trouble breathing. She told him, flatly and without emotion, that she needed to go to the emergency room.

■   ■   ■

That same Thursday, a cool and overcast one in the South Bay, Governor Gavin Newsom shut down California. Executive Order N-33-20 urged the state's 40 million people to stay home, making the state the first in the country to experience a full clampdown on normal life. It wouldn't be the last. Illinois and New Jersey followed two days later. Then New York. Then Connecticut, Louisiana, Ohio, Oregon, and Washington. By the time the month was out, three-fourths of Americans, 245 million people, were being told not to leave home except to perform essential jobs or to fill their own critical needs for food and medical care. Looser versions of the authoritarian lockdown measures pioneered in China were chasing the virus throughout the United States.

California shuttered itself at a time when the state was reporting 675 cases and 16 deaths, though testing problems meant no one knew what the real number was. Newsom cited alarming projections that more than half the state could get infected in the next two months—at least 25 million people. The point of the shutdown, he explained, was to ward off those infections and make the projections "moot." He said he had faith that Californians would abide by the restrictions to protect each other. "There is a social contract here," he said. "People, I think, recognize the need to do more and to meet this moment."

What Huy recognized was that his mom needed urgent medical care, one of few permissible reasons to leave the house and few ways to get her off the couch. He guided her into the car and aimed it at the Kaiser Permanente hospital in Santa Clara while she tried, weary and unwell, to keep resting. She wasn't the type to betray worry about having to race to the ER even while a deadly pandemic had mostly emptied the streets that led there. But Huy could tell she was struggling. It wasn't until he slid into a parking spot, stepped out of the car, and started steering his mother toward the hospital entrance that he noticed just how slowly she was moving.

Hospital staffers were standing outside the doors, blocking

them to keep the number of entrants restricted. Huy stood before them with his mom as she struggled for breath, explaining why she needed to be allowed inside. When she was finally permitted to plod through the sliding doors and Huy moved to accompany her, he found his entrance barred. No one can go into the waiting room but the patient, he was told. Too risky.

Liên was already making her way inside. Watching her shuffle away from him, knowing she was suffering and powerless even just to keep her company, let alone soothe her, he told himself she was only going to be in the hospital for a few days, at the end of which she'd be feeling much better. He hadn't given her a parting hug; he just shouted goodbye from the sidewalk—said he'd call her later and that he'd be back soon to take her home again.

As he drove away, he could already feel a sickness surfacing in his own body. His muscles were beginning to ache. It stood to reason, he supposed; if his mom had the flu, he'd probably caught it. He didn't seriously entertain the idea it might be something worse until his mom called from the hospital the next day.

She'd gotten a Covid test. It had come back positive.

■   ■   ■

No one knew how, exactly, the virus had wandered into Liên's airways. Perhaps it was at that last housewarming party Liên had attended with Nghề, where the hosts later turned out to have been infected. Regardless, even as she had puttered about the house and prepared for a few days of babysitting her little grandson, the tiny invader had been settling into soft membranes in her nose and throat, stabbing into healthy cells with its protein spikes, forcing its genes inside, and turning Liên's own cells into mini-manufacturers of more virus, pumping out an arsenal of little deadly weapons that would turn Liên's lungs into a battle zone.

Lungs are miraculous, delicate things, sitting in everybody's chest cavity, quietly doing the business of keeping them alive by pulling oxygen from the air and delivering it to the blood. They are short in the front, reaching midway down the chest, and longer in the back, like a mullet or a Jazz Age tuxedo jacket. Threaded through their spongy tissue are tunnels that split and subdivide until they become thousands of tiny pathways that dead-end into millions of fragile little air sacs, with linings so thin that oxygen molecules can pass through into the mesh of small blood vessels that surround them. They then collect the blood cells' carbon dioxide waste to be pushed out of the body on the exhale.

If the body's immune system didn't halt the new coronavirus in time, viral legions could advance from the nose and throat and into the lungs, killing cells that line the upper airways and littering those passages with detritus, making it difficult to breathe. Meanwhile, as the body dispatched immune-cell reinforcements to try to neutralize the invader, the immune cells themselves caused inflammation in the lungs and further compromised breathing. Sometimes the virus hordes advanced yet further, into the little air sacs at the boundary with the blood. Here was where the body's own frantic efforts to save itself could wind up destroying it instead, as inflammation filled the air sacs and blocked the life-sustaining transfer of oxygen into blood cells. In some instances, the delicate bulbs could be so damaged that fluid started to spill into the lungs from the surrounding blood vessels, a condition known as acute respiratory distress syndrome. Once this threshold was crossed, a Covid patient was unlikely to survive.

But the virus known as SARS-CoV-2 exhibited a range of other behaviors as well, and a baffling variety of outcomes for the infected. You could be infected and show no symptoms at all. You could mysteriously lose your sense of taste or smell; experience nausea, vomiting, or diarrhea; develop rashes or foot lesions known as "Covid toes"; or, in the worst cases, experience organ damage beyond the lungs, including to the heart and the brain. The same little bundle of genes and protein could have no effect on one person and kill another.

After Liên's positive test, Huy and his sister finally started to freak out; their mom was in danger, and the whole family was exposed. The Les rushed to get tests themselves. Huy's father got one: positive. Uyên back in Nevada got one: positive.

Huy got one: negative.

The result made no sense to him. He was surrounded by Covid at home, and his symptoms were only getting worse. In fact, he was finding it hard to breathe.

The Vaccine Developer

The Gamble

January 7–January 23, 2020

B<small>Y THE TIME</small> H<small>UY'S FAMILY</small> members knew they were sick, a young stranger on the other side of the country had already spent months racing for a remedy, obsessed with preventing others from catching the illness. The battle against the new coronavirus had consumed her long before the Les understood its threat, and in fact, when the Les were diagnosed mid-March, she already had an experimental formula for an inoculation shot. She'd spend the remainder of the year trying to prove it worked, with the entire world depending on her largely anonymous efforts. And her odyssey started in the most banal of ways, with an email.

It came on a bleak winter Tuesday. At around 8:30 a.m. on that January 7, when her CEO showed up in her inbox, Hamilton Bennett was already at her desk at Moderna, which was really her patch of a long table in the open-concept office, where a whiteboard half-wall divided off the workspaces on the other side. Hamilton's desk-mate had markered a counter on its surface to track the days since

Hamilton's Subaru had last broken down and kept having to reset the counter to zero.

Stephane Bancel, the CEO, was promiscuous with his emails, fond of firing off one-line missives even to subordinates way below him on the corporate food chain as questions or ideas popped into his brain. Often he'd be wondering about something he'd heard in a meeting—*What's going on with this?*—and it wasn't unusual for Hamilton, who was a program manager running vaccine development, to get pulled into frantic hours-long email conversations trying to hunt down the information he wanted.

In this case, clicking in, Hamilton saw an exchange begun earlier that morning between Stephane and one of Moderna's collaborators at the National Institutes of Health. A *Wall Street Journal* article on January 6 had described medical officials in China "racing to identify the cause of a mystery viral pneumonia" that, at least according to Chinese authorities, had already infected nearly 60 people and put seven into critical condition. Stephane had written to Barney Graham, the deputy director of the Vaccine Research Center at the National Institute of Allergy and Infectious Diseases (NIAID). Did anyone know what this new virus was? Barney wrote back: he did not. But it might be a coronavirus. That, in a strange way, could be good news.

Hamilton herself knew little about the new outbreak. Major American newspapers had just begun tracking the spread of a strange respiratory illness that seemed to be linked to a seafood and wild-animal market in Wuhan, a city of 11 million in central China. Hong Kong and Singapore were issuing health alerts. Reports recited statistics about prior twenty-first century respiratory disease epidemics: SARS, or severe acute respiratory syndrome, had been identified in China; had infected more than 8,000 people across 30 countries and killed more than 700 between 2002 and 2003; and then had apparently burned itself out after about 9 months. MERS, or Middle East respiratory syndrome, had been discovered in Saudi Arabia a decade later and never entirely disappeared; had similarly spread widely, to 27 countries; and had yielded a higher overall death toll of 881 among 2,562 cases confirmed—making it a deadlier but less contagious disease.

Both were cousins in the same viral family, other members of which could produce the runny noses and coughing fits of the common cold. But Chinese authorities had ruled out either as the cause of the new outbreak, which some suggested was really nothing to worry about. One former public health official in China was so confident in the country's infection-control advances since the SARS outbreak that he assured the *Washington Post*, "It's impossible for something like SARS to happen again." Still, if the disease turned out to be caused by a coronavirus like those other two outbreaks, Barney believed that Moderna had a chance to prove itself.

Which the company needed, because so far its revolutionary promise—that you could hijack human cells' own machinery to make vaccines at record speeds—had gotten it billions in investments but hadn't produced a single approved drug in its entire decade of existence.

The idea was as simple as it was devilishly difficult to execute: The company would fashion medicines from messenger RNA (mRNA), the genetic recipes that cells naturally used to whip up the proteins the body depends on for all kinds of functions—including powering the immune system. The right mRNA sequence could instruct a cell to make any kind of disease-fighting protein a person could think of, sidestepping time-consuming lab manufacturing in favor of using evolution's own proven processes, and in effect, as the biotech reporter Damian Garde put it, transforming "human cells into drug factories." Moderna executives evangelized the approach's virtues for diseases as varied as diabetes and cancer, and its potential to usher in a future of bespoke medicines tailored to each individual. In the company's early years, it raised a lot of money, published no data, and developed a reputation for secrecy as much as swagger.

Because it really wasn't clear, for all the hype and mystique surrounding Moderna, that the technology could work. The problem was that mRNA was unstable, meant to stick around long enough to deliver its instructions to cells' protein-making machinery and then disintegrate. Introducing foreign mRNA into someone's body might actually be worse than useless—the person's immune system could attack and destroy the invader before it even made a delivery to a target cell, generating side effects that could hurt the patient in the process. For these reasons, even though researchers had been exploring mRNA's promise since the mid-1990s, major pharmaceutical companies had largely given up on working with it. Moderna itself, a few years into its existence, had shifted focus from the flashiest possibilities to a modest suite of vaccine candidates.

But Hamilton was a true believer. In fact, at the time she scanned that fateful email chain on January 7, she already had a call on the books with Barney of the Vaccine Research Center for later in the week to discuss an ambitious experiment. The prior fall,

Stephane had wagered Barney's team that Moderna's newest factory could produce a new vaccine in just 60 days. This didn't count the time needed to conduct trials and get regulatory approval, but it was still an audacious feat. The record for fastest-licensed inoculation was held by the mumps vaccine, which had taken four years to get developed and approved by the Food and Drug Administration (FDA). The same process for the rotavirus vaccine had taken more than two decades. Most vaccines failed in development. But Stephane was so confident in his company's manufacturing plant that he had planned a test to show just how quickly Moderna could produce a trial-ready vaccine: All they needed was to pick a virus.

Maybe this new one in China was it.

■   ■   ■

A professor had once told Hamilton that he'd never encourage his children to go into science, because the lows were really low and the highs were just all right. Hamilton, a bleeding-heart public-health enthusiast and a sweet-speaking compulsive achiever, got it instinctively. She'd grown up in part on a Kentucky hay farm, fox hunting for fun: a sport in which, in the United States at least, many hunters ride horses around and never actually catch a fox. Science could feel much the same way. "You spend your life working towards something and no one else is ever going to understand what it took to get there or the importance of what you think is incredible," she explained. "To you, it feels amazing. And then you realize no one else understands and it just like, knocks you down a peg."

As if to test the professor's theory, she chased the kinds of work least likely to offer glory or money. She once tried to convince her husband to move with her to Sri Lanka so she could study water filtration. (He declined, and they opted to live closer to his family on the East Coast.) But her true passion was emerging infectious diseases. She'd caught the bug, so to speak, during a high school internship at a Boston hospital. A patient would come in with symptoms, and an infectious disease specialist would launch his own mini-*CSI* to root out the cause. Once a man came in with a rash and dark circles on his lower legs, and the doctor eventually traced the ailment back to a golfing trip in Connecticut, identifying a case of Lyme disease that labs had missed.

She spent a few years on the Boston biotech scene working on exotic-sounding products such as small-molecule inhibitors and monoclonal antibodies. But in 2016, when an outbreak of the mosquito-borne Zika virus was spreading through Brazil and out to other countries, Hamilton wanted to help fix it. The disease didn't manifest in symptoms for most patients, but it saved its harshest cruelty for the next generation. Women infected during pregnancy could find their newborns arriving with small heads and brain damage or even partially collapsed skulls, resulting in developmental difficulties destined to last a lifetime—if those children even survived.

Hamilton had meanwhile heard of a plucky startup in Kendall Square that was making bold promises to "disrupt" the drug industry as the world knew it, using the still-unproven magic of mRNA. And it had won a multimillion-dollar government contract, through the Biomedical Advanced Research and Development Authority (BARDA), to develop a Zika vaccine. She'd never worked on a vaccine before, but she had run BARDA-funded projects, so she pushed out her resume to anyone she knew with any connection to Moderna, and hoped for a phone call.

She got the call, she interviewed, she heard entrancing ideas about mRNA's possibilities, and one of her interviewers even signed her up for an obscure newsletter he thought she'd be interested in, focused on vaccines for possible epidemics. She was wowed by the technology and touched by the gesture. Emerging infectious diseases is a largely thankless field, where the commercial incentives don't always align with the value of saving lives. It's tough to make a profit by plowing money into decades' worth of research and development to prevent or cure diseases in poor countries. But if the process could be streamlined with mRNA—made faster, more precise, cheaper—you could stop worrying as much about how to make money and focus on a different set of questions: Where are the unmet needs? What can this technology do?

The man who would become her boss told her about a combo vaccine he wanted to make for tropical diseases, to immunize against yellow fever, dengue, Zika, and chikungunya all in one shot. From there you could think through all kinds of science-fiction scenarios, tailor combo vaccines for a traveler on the basis of the countries she was visiting, or combine all the childhood vaccinations into two shots versus four or six.

And then, if you could perfect the process enough, get it to the point where you could keep various prototype mRNAs in the freezer and just take them out to whip up into vaccine form as needed, you could put the technology in hospitals all over the world. You could have the vaccine technology sitting at a hospital in China. And if there was an outbreak, you could track down those infected, trace their contacts, and within a few days make a vaccine on demand to inoculate everyone who'd been exposed, rather than wait for it to become a pandemic.

A Zika vaccine might help the company get there.

Production of vaccines typically required growing a virus or other pathogen in a lab, weakening or deactivating it, then delivering it into human cells. The immune system of the injected human in question would then, if the vaccine worked, produce antibodies, protein weapons that could block and disarm the dummy pathogen and summon other immune warriors to come and destroy it. Thus equipped and trained against a practice opponent, the immune system would be ready when it encountered the very similar real one.

The mRNA approach cut out a step—you didn't have to, say, grow a flu virus in a chicken egg and then manipulate it into a safe form. You could give a person's cells the instructions to make their own harmless bits of virus as rehearsal sparring partners for the immune system.

This also meant you could get a vaccine on a much faster timeline than what the industry was accustomed to. With Zika spreading fast in 2016, Hamilton hoped the method might be a chance to stop it fast, too.

She got the job at a time when multiple other companies were also pursuing a vaccine, as the disease cascaded through some 70 countries. Unlike some other tropical diseases, this one was coming to rich countries, which meant there were suddenly dollars available for research and development, and a potentially big market for whichever company won the race. Researchers were foretelling an outrageous pace of just two years to get the vaccine to market, slicing the existing speed record in half. The head of the NIAID, Anthony Fauci, ordered "all hands on deck" and told the *New York Times* that most people in the field were confident about getting a vaccine.

Hamilton's Zika program was the fastest vaccine program yet for Moderna, racing from getting the genetic sequence of the virus to the first clinical trials—which is to say, human testing—in just 10 months. (Inovio Pharmaceuticals went even faster with its DNA-based vaccine, setting a record by launching trials in a mere eight months.)

But eight months into Moderna's clinical trials, when Hamilton and the team started to get results back, they found that their vaccine candidate wasn't generating a strong enough immune response to protect people from the virus. Hamilton combed back through the process, trying to puzzle out what had happened—was the manufacturing faulty somehow?—and finally discovered that the viral sequence her team had been using as the basis of the entire project contained errors. Basically, a genetic typo. So that was 18 months of sprinting for a vaccine only to wind up back at the starting line.

The lows are really low.

Hamilton didn't tend to react emotionally to failures like this, which might have made another person's stomach drop. Part of the point, however, had been to be fast, and by the time the team got a new vaccine formula into clinical trials, the Zika virus had slipped out of the headlines. It continued to spread, though not with its 2016 fervor—which in turn made vaccine testing difficult, because tests required subjects getting exposed to the disease in order to prove that the vaccine could protect them. It was 2020 before the team

started to see new results from the first phase of human testing, and
by then, the world was wrestling with a far deadlier epidemic.

■   ■   ■

Hamilton had meanwhile been cooking up ways to speed the manufacture of vaccines for emerging infectious diseases, with the hope
of creating a vault of potential vaccines that could be rapidly tested
and deployed in case of an outbreak. The idea was to take a given
virus, like a pandemic influenza virus or a Lassa virus or a Nipah
virus—something that most of the time you didn't have to worry
about, but that had the potential to become a major threat—and
begin the vaccine-making process proactively: develop the product,
start early trials in animals and safety tests in humans, and be ready
to pull an inoculation off the shelf for final trials and approval if
the disease did break out in force. No epidemic, no problem: You
wouldn't have wasted resources on enormous efficacy studies involving thousands of people. But you'd have made small bets against a
number of different, unlikely but potentially catastrophic outbreaks,
which (a) gave you a six-month head start on a fully tested and
approved vaccine in case of an actual epidemic, and (b) significantly
raised the chances of, one day, literally saving the world.

She'd been having discussions about this with various government actors—at NIAID, at the Defense Department, at BARDA—
to get ideas and to find funding. This was why she had that call
scheduled with Barney Graham in the second week of January, and
why the new virus circulating in China looked like it might be a
good candidate, especially because it was spreading even as she
checked her email.

By Thursday, January 9, Chinese authorities had identified a new kind of coronavirus as the culprit for the outbreak. This confirmed Barney's earlier hunch, which was useful, because it also happened that NIAID scientists had already studied the coronavirus family during the SARS and MERS outbreaks. In the SARS case, it had taken them around 20 months to get their vaccine candidate ready to test in humans, by which point they'd missed the outbreak. A MERS vaccine that NIAID and Moderna had collaborated on was still only in the research phase eight years after MERS first showed up. Still, by now scientists at both Moderna and NIAID knew a lot about coronaviruses, how they attacked human cells, and what it might take to stop them.

A potential complication was that this coronavirus outbreak might burn itself out even more quickly than the previous two. By the time Chinese scientists had pinpointed the type of pathogen responsible, authorities hadn't confirmed any new cases at the epicenter for about two weeks. One researcher speculated to the *Washington Post* that because the Huanan Seafood Wholesale Market linked to many sicknesses had shut down, the disease might simply go away.

Nevertheless, during their phone call on Friday, January 10, Hamilton and Barney agreed to start trying to find a vaccine for the new virus; the genetic sequence should become public within days, at which point Moderna and NIAID scientists could work to design the vaccine formula. Moderna's manufacturers could then kick off their sprint to a product, and NIAID, with its well-developed research infrastructure, could run the lab experiments on animals and the first phase of clinical trials in people. In fact, on that same Friday, a consortium of Chinese scientists published a draft of the needed sequence, a document that looked like a mish-mash of the same four letters in different orders, 30,000-odd letters long: "attaaaggtt tataccttcc caggtaacaa."

In there somewhere, buried in the virus's own genes, lurked the key to its demise.

But that same weekend, on Saturday, January 11, Chinese officials also reported for the first time that the disease the virus caused had killed a person.

■   ■   ■

Hamilton now had an approximate mug shot of the killer. The virus's outer membrane had a coat of spikes that to some scientists brought to mind the points on a crown, hence the term *corona-virus*. Actually, up close, the surface looked more like a field of broccoli stalks, and a very weird one at that, because the broccoli didn't stay in one place. It waved about and wandered around the outer membrane, confusing the host's immune system with its shape-shifting. The spikes were what the virus used to fasten onto a host cell and then slurp its own genetic material inside and create a clone army of itself.

Hamilton knew from the SARS experience that if you could block the spike, you would in effect block the entire virus. In immune system terms, you'd want an antibody to stick itself to the spike and prevent it from attaching itself to a cell.

Now the genome was public, and within that very long string of letters were the genetic instructions for the spike. Hamilton would have to get Moderna's research team to locate those instructions and then back-engineer the mRNA recipe that told human cells how to make the spike themselves. That would be the basis for a vaccine: The cells would learn to produce the spike, and the immune system would generate the antibodies to disable it, without ever encountering the real virus. Then the person's immune system would be ready to meet and neutralize a coronavirus invader if it came.

Having alerted the research scientists to what was needed, Hamilton spent the weekend mentally tapping her foot. The team knew what protein spikes looked like genetically; it shouldn't take that long to find and isolate the right sequence. Where was it? Hamilton kept texting one of the scientists. Why was it taking so long?

When it finally arrived on Monday, Hamilton immediately spotted a problem—she had before her a sequence more than a thousand letters long that would be the longest mRNA strand Moderna had ever tested in people. The longer the sequence, the more opportunities there were for mistakes, for breaks, for difficulty manufacturing: in short, for failure. Meanwhile, the manufacturing team was promising it could put together a product by April, a timeline that also sounded crazy to her, given her record-setting 10-month dash to a Zika vaccine just a few years before.

But she had a safeguard against the Zika experience, and the initial failure of the vaccine she'd tried to develop. Her NIAID collaborators had made their own attempt to design the vaccine and came up with the exact same sequence. This was independent corroboration they were on the right track.

Now she just had to convince her bosses to divert resources for the sake of an experiment on a virus that still hadn't hit U.S. shores, and, for all she knew, might go away in a few months.

Yet the world was about to shift.

Researchers at Johns Hopkins University in Baltimore were tracking the virus as it spread from China and into South Korea and Japan. A Chinese civil-engineering PhD student, Ensheng Dong, had been hearing updates about infections from family back home and watching a harrowing story unfold in the official statistics. At the encouragement of a faculty adviser, he launched a Web dashboard and map to track cases of the new disease.

The site soon became a must-check resource for people concerned about the spread of the new coronavirus, be they journalists or researchers or ordinary citizens looking for some way to understand the strange new disaster starting to enfold Asia. Hamilton kept refreshing the Web page, watching the red dots of contagion grow into blobs that oozed their way across larger and larger sections of the map. And then, on January 21, a dot bloomed in Seattle.

Hamilton started to think maybe the vaccine project wasn't just a drill.

Two days later, on her 35th birthday, she showed up in one of Moderna's conference rooms, on time for a meeting of the company's executive committee, including CEO Stephane Bancel and President Stephen Hoge. Stephane was a stickler for meeting punctuality, and despite his being in Davos for the World Economic Forum, his voice was there on schedule, piping through the speakerphone with bad sound as he walked between buildings. Stephen was nowhere in sight yet, though Hamilton knew he was going to take some convincing.

Stephen was the one who led research and development, planned the pipelines, and made sure the company was developing the right products. He had plans for 2020; he was trying get rare disease programs up and running; he was trying to start the company's first large clinical study, of a vaccine for cytomegalovirus (CMV); the company needed to do another round of fundraising if they were even going to take the CMV vaccine into final, large-scale trials, let alone operate for the next three to five years. Stephane was already convinced this new virus was going to be huge: He'd told Stephen as much in early January, calling him, worked up, from Europe at around 4:00 a.m. Boston time, while Stephen just tried to drink his coffee in the living room. It was all well and good for Stephane to have an amazing vision, but Stephen was going to have to figure out how to make it work, and he didn't want to go chasing some shiny object.

And now Hamilton was prepared to tell him she wanted to seize resources, maybe even kick a program out of his pipeline, and reallocate those resources to a pilot program with her in charge.

But Stephen was running late, and Stephane was on her side, and it wasn't the first time he'd been her partner in crime to push for more work on infectious diseases. Plus, he was growing more and more alarmed by what he was seeing out of China, how quickly the virus was spreading there and popping up elsewhere. Even though he sympathized with the worry that a coronavirus vaccine could distract from other work Moderna was trying to do—well, why couldn't they do all of it? Hamilton had in fact been doing all of it since early January, dealing with her normal substantial work-load keeping the Zika program on track while also trying to hustle a Covid vaccine into production, secure grants, find partners for trials, map out timelines.

She spent the bulk of her days until 5:00 p.m. reviewing the data coming in for the Zika vaccine and planning for its next phase of clinical trials. Then she'd spend hours, sometimes until 10 at night, combing through all the emails she'd missed during the day about the fledgling Covid vaccine program, collating that day's progress in research or manufacturing, setting priorities, planning next steps.

She launched into her proposal, describing the players and responsibilities, as well as her hopes they could start the first phase of clinical trials by April or, more conservatively, May. Stephane didn't have much critical feedback to offer; it all sounded fine to him. By the time Stephen showed up about 10 minutes into the meeting, Stephane had already approved the program. Stephen knew that even if he really wanted to stop them, he stood as much of a chance as a crossing guard holding up a stop sign in front of a freight train. He also knew that Hamilton could strategize a way around any operational objection he put in front of her. And if there simply weren't enough people at the company to do the job, she'd convince others to work twice as hard while she worked four times as hard.

Later that day, Hamilton took a rare break from work for her birthday, to go get dinner with her husband at a new chicken place that had opened up. She was a sucker for southern fried chicken. She didn't know she wouldn't be going to restaurants for very much longer.

The CEO

Ramping Up

WHILE HAMILTON WORRIED about preventing Covid, Chris Kiple worried about what happened when someone already had it so bad they couldn't breathe. On March 12, he was hopping between hot spots trying to solve this problem. The World Health Organization had just declared the Covid crisis a pandemic, New York City had declared a state of emergency, and Chris, the young CEO of a small ventilator company called Ventec, based outside Seattle, was suddenly facing a level of demand he'd never seen before. He had just wrapped up a meeting in New York, where officials overseeing the state's ventilator stockpile had discussed with him some terrifying possibilities—including that the state could soon face a shortage of tens of thousands of machines, though it could be a lot more or a lot less, no one could say for certain. Chris was among few people anywhere who could help, and he hadn't been able to offer much but information—his factory, one of only a handful in the world that manufactured ventilators, could only produce about 200 a month. As he boarded a plane back home to Washington State, he was scared and discouraged.

And though New York was getting hit the hardest with the disease, Chris's own state had gotten hit first. On January 21, the CDC had announced what it then believed to be the only Covid case in the United States, afflicting a man in his thirties in Snohomish County, a heavily wooded patch of northern Washington State. The patient had flown, symptom-free, from a family visit at the outbreak's center in Wuhan, China, and arrived at Seattle–Tacoma International Airport on January 15. He began to show symptoms a day later and wound up in a medical isolation unit that week. A county health official said there probably wasn't much risk to the public. Meanwhile China's outbreak, if you trusted the official statistics, still involved a few hundred cases, and a single-digit death toll.

President Trump shut down most travel from China in late January, some two weeks after that first confirmation of a U.S. case imported from there, and the government evacuated hundreds of Americans from the country and put them under a two-week federal quarantine at various military bases. The Snohomish patient recovered. And an outbreak gathered force at a nursing home not far away, in Kirkland, Washington.

Kirkland was the home of the bulk-and-bargain store COSTCO's first corporate headquarters and the name it affixed to its store brand—you could get Kirkland Signature olive oil, cat food, quinoa, jugs of bourbon. It was also the site of the Evergreen Hospital, where, on February 29, Washington state health officials and the CDC announced what was then the first known U.S. Covid death. That same hospital was turning into a receiving station for elderly residents of the nearby Life Care Center of Kirkland, some of them checking in with severe respiratory symptoms. A woman in her seventies showed up with breathing trouble, a 103-degree fever, and low oxygen; was placed on a ventilator; and died within a week, on March 2.

This was happening just a few miles down the 405 from Ventec's Bothell headquarters, where Chris worked, and it kept happening, turning the Life Care Center into America's first known hot spot. Frantic investigations into the cluster of respiratory illnesses, which had at first looked like the flu, yielded a count of 142 COVID-19 cases among residents, staff, and visitors. By mid-March, the nursing home had been linked to a quarter of Covid fatalities nationwide. The disease ultimately killed 39 of about 120 Life Care Center residents.

The outbreak was a harbinger of the particular dangers Covid posed to the elderly, and in nursing homes specifically. In the first few months of the pandemic, more than 40 percent of Covid deaths were tied to nursing homes, the disease killing either their residents or their employees. Many such facilities nationwide already exhibited poor infection control—with a highly contagious disease that preyed on the elderly, at a moment when testing, protective equipment, and even basic knowledge about the disease were scarce, they didn't stand a chance.

Chris's flight from New York stopped on a layover, and he was killing time in Houston when his cell phone rang. Someone from the Washington governor's office was on the line, on behalf of another state government scrambling for resources and unsure where to turn. Chris was fresh off explaining the basics of ventilator manufacturing to one set of officials, and here came another with just as little grasp on the basic problem the state was facing. The governor's aide couldn't understand why, as the state was getting hit with Covid and anticipated needing ventilators, ventilators were becoming impossible to get. Weren't these just machines that blew air? Why was this so hard?

Chris tried to explain. Ventilators were complex instruments. His company's own small machine, which just looked like a plastic box with a screen and some buttons, about the size of a toaster oven laid on its side, was made up of 700 parts from more than a hundred different suppliers. All of those suppliers had spent months getting overwhelmed with orders before the U.S. even started really thinking about the problem. China wanted the same things while the virus pummeled the country in January and February, ditto Italy as Covid's fury shifted there in February and early March. By the time Chris landed in Houston, those countries and others had already been ordering ventilators by the thousands and were still experiencing shortages in some cases. Even as Chris took the call from Washington, doctors in Italy had started rationing ventilators on the basis of who was most likely to survive, which often meant that the most vulnerable patients were left to die.

The United States was months behind in this scramble. Ventec executives had sent emails to the CDC as early as February, offering to help, but at that point the federal government barely knew how to react or what kind of help would really be needed. In the interim, U.S. companies had slid far down the purchase-order queues for things like blowers and circuit boards that were necessary to get air pumping through the machines properly. Even if Ventec, with its

130 or so employees, were to go on a hiring spree and drive all those employees to exhaustion chasing impossible production targets, it would be useless without having the proper parts to put together, many of which were being completely consumed elsewhere.

Chris got off the phone, flew home, and went directly to the office, where he worked into the early morning of Friday, March 13, before snatching a few hours of sleep and then plunging back into the storm.

Which, that day, exploded into a hurricane.

The president declared the Covid outbreak a national emergency. Frantic calls poured in to the Ventec offices. They seemed to come from everywhere. Hospital administrators, governors, foreign heads of state. Chris could hear the panic in their voices. Everyone saw what was happening in China and Italy; the U.S. national emergency only confirmed what so many already knew. Hospitals in hard-hit countries were already running out of the simple ways to defend the caretakers: masks, gowns, gloves. And once the virus got past that first line of defense, it was that much harder to beat. One article in the *New England Journal of Medicine* argued that even though protective-equipment shortages could prove deadly over time, the absence of a needed breathing machine could kill a person on the spot. "When patients' breathing deteriorates to the point that they need a ventilator," the authors wrote, "there is typically only a limited window during which they can be saved. And when the machine is withdrawn from patients who are fully ventilator-dependent, they will usually die within minutes." In a single day, by Chris's estimate, his company went from having about 200 ventilators in stock to about a thousand on back order. And the calls kept coming.

The crisis still had yet to fully hit the United States on that Friday, but it was obvious which way the trend was going. The virus was moving through the population faster than anyone could track it, but the shaky official count stood around 2,000 cases, spread through nearly every state, with 47 deaths. The real count was certainly much higher, but even this underestimate via sparse tests showed about a 133-fold explosion in cases from just the month before, on February 13, when the CDC had confirmed America's 15th known infection. "There will likely be additional cases in the coming days and weeks," the agency's press release had predicted mildly at the time.

Now desperate caretakers and decision makers, who could easily see the fearsome future bearing down on them and were largely powerless to help, kept turning to Chris and finding that he was largely powerless, too. Hospitals needed to prepare; they needed ventilators tomorrow, this weekend. Ventec didn't have any left and couldn't move fast enough to save the lives that would be at risk in the coming months. It was a terrible feeling, wanting to help, being asked for help, and having to tell desperate people: *We can't.*

Especially because Chris knew that practically no one else could, either. There were perhaps 12 manufacturers worldwide capable of making critical-care ventilators, several based overseas and focused on filling orders from their own countries or other places that had asked first, overcommitted and with nothing left for the United States. If everyone else was tapped out, Ventec was it.

■   ■   ■

Chris did not present as the type of person susceptible to being overwhelmed. He had the upbeat, let's-go-change-the-world affect of the serial entrepreneur that he was, and the polished swagger of the attorney and investment banker that he had been. He was a blandly handsome, hair-slicked-back, hard-charging executive type you could picture wearing sweatervests in elementary school, except midwestern nice from a Nebraska upbringing; he liked to talk about "thinking outside the box," and the only social media he really used was LinkedIn. He'd moved, improbably, into ventilator sales at the behest of a mentor, leaving investment banking behind because he liked the idea of spending his time concretely making people's lives better. He knew, to some degree, the struggles of having a severely ill family member. One of his two older brothers—Chris was the youngest of four siblings, also including a sister—suffered from a muscular degenerative condition that made breathing difficult during sleep and some other activities. Years after Chris joined Ventec, his brother started using one of its ventilators for help.

Chris was on the sales side when he joined the company, in which capacity he'd stay in the homes of ventilator-dependent patients and their families or in long-term care facilities, asking people questions, watching them operate the devices, trying to understand their problems and how to improve Ventec's device to make a very difficult lifestyle a little bit easier. Because no one wanted to end up on a ventilator, and no one expected it. You could wake up one day feeling perfectly healthy, and then get in a car accident, injure your spinal cord while diving, get a diagnosis of a muscular or neurodegenerative disease such as amyotrophic lateral sclerosis (ALS), also known as Lou Gehrig's disease. Your child could be born prematurely and require one of the machines to survive.

For Covid patients, being intubated on a ventilator in most cases meant lying sedated on a hospital bed, the machine keeping the breath going via a tube through the windpipe, so that the body could stay alive long enough to defeat the infection. Some patients spent weeks this way. The longer the treatment went on, the lower the chances of survival and the more difficult the recovery period, due not least to the toll of prolonged sedation. But if the patient recovered, in most cases that individual would return to breathing on his or her own.

Other, chronic conditions such as ALS could require long-term ventilation, lasting years or decades. Certain portable devices could aid the breathing through a mask or nasal tubes or, more invasively, with a tube inserted into the windpipe through an incision in the throat. This meant a ventilator-dependent patient could potentially live at home, maybe walk, have sex, enjoy some attributes of normal life even without being able to breathe independently. The physicist Stephen Hawking had lived with ALS and on a ventilator for decades. Hawking had been dead two years when the pandemic hit, and his family wound up donating his ventilator to the Cambridge hospital that had treated him, to assist them in fighting COVID-19.

It was the long-term patients that Chris first focused on when he joined Ventec, and he did everything with some of them, even to the point of accompanying them to a public bathroom and noticing how the bacteria filter made a wheelchair-mounted device too big to wedge into a stall. He watched one patient, after Ventec designed a smaller filter, finally maneuver the chair and machine through the swinging door without getting stuck, and saw the patient's family members cry with relief and joy over the simple act of being able to use a public restroom. Another time a mother called him up to say she'd been able to go out for coffee with her ventilator-dependent son. A trip to a bathroom or to a Starbucks—these were such ordinary events that, for some, could seem hopelessly out of reach. And then, because of a ventilator, a patient could grasp on to a richer life.

Chris found it moving, and not just because of the patients. A ventilator dependency within a household affected everyone in it. The person needing ventilation often depended on caregivers for basic tasks, including eating, drinking, and visiting the toilet. Anything that made the therapy easier and more efficient, kept the patient out of the hospital, reduced the overall anxiety of having a loved one with such a severe illness, could change life for the whole family. A parent might have more time to spend with their other kids or be able to go back to work.

But fundamentally, Chris was helping to manage a relatively rare problem for a niche client base. Ventilators were so specialized, and so far from most people's minds, that no one even kept track of how many or which kinds were in the country, scattered among homes, hospitals, and state and national stockpiles. Someone had made an attempt to count in 2009, finding about 60,000 full-featured ventilators in hospitals, and maybe 100,000 simpler models, not necessarily intended for critical patients, that could be used in a pinch. Few people needed to know this or had reason to suspect that a devastating respiratory pandemic was lurking at the end of the next decade.

Now, in 2020, five years into Chris's tenure at Ventec, after he'd worked his way rapidly from sales to chief operating officer to president to CEO, ventilators were not simply a matter of easing individual and family struggle. They were at the center of a national emergency.

■ ■ ■

If no one really knew how many ventilators were in the United States in March 2020 to begin with—an oft-cited guess, extrapolating from that 2009 survey, was around 200,000—still less could anyone predict how many the country would need to help treat a disease whose course was still wildly uncertain. Projected Covid death tolls careened from one extreme to another. One horrifying study released by Imperial College London on March 16 calculated that, in the unlikely absence of any mitigating measures at all, the disease could kill 2.2 million people in the United States alone. The White House embraced a more cheerful model predicting around 80,000 American deaths from the disease by August.

Estimates of America's ventilator need were similarly wide-ranging: tens of thousands, half a million, close to a million. The nationwide shortfall could be in the hundreds of thousands. Chris estimated that, worldwide, ventilator manufacturers could probably produce about 40,000 to 50,000 units a year, which wouldn't come close to meeting the anticipated shortfall in the United States—and Germany had just ordered 10,000, wiping out at a stroke a fifth of what the world could produce in the next 12 months. Ventec, making at most a couple hundred machines a month, barely stood to make a dent.

Chris knew two things: First, that the company had to do more, had to max out its staff and its money and its parts suppliers completely and make as many ventilators as possible. Second, that it wouldn't be enough.

Still, there was no other option but to try to help save as many people as possible. Chris figured the absolute most the team could do in the short term with the resources available was quintuple its output, to 1,000 machines a month. Even that ambition, pitifully insignificant to the crisis as it seemed, stretched the limits of difficulty till it touched crazy.

Indeed, what Chris got from much of his team in the days after his New York trip when he presented this idea, as expressed via polite corporate euphemism, was "pushback." More starkly, certain colleagues thought he was nuts, and told him repeatedly it would be impossible. There weren't enough people at the company; they'd need to go on a hiring spree and organize shifts to keep the factory running 24 hours a day. They needed more space for the new hires, for the workstations to assemble small parts into subassemblies—metering valves, compressors, cough assists. Plus enough space to make sure the factory workers could stay a safe six feet apart. And then more space for all the testing stations, to make sure each individual subassembly worked as it was supposed to, before putting all those pieces on the center band and then, finally, testing the whole thing again. The company had no experience operating on the scale Chris now envisioned.

That was actually the easy part. The nearly insurmountable part—was parts. Maybe you could man a factory, but it took more than that to make a ventilator—you needed circuit boards, blower motors, plastic tubes, touch-screens, casings, buttons. Ventec was nowhere near the biggest player in the ventilator market, and nowhere near the top priority for manufacturers backlogged with orders. Having historically ordered maybe a few dozen parts a month from any given supplier, the company would now be attempting to order thousands a month, or even millions. And it was, not coincidentally, the middle of a pandemic. Many factories were shutting down and sending workers home. Ventec wasn't sitting on the cash reserves of the bigger players such as Medtronic and Philips. Was the company really in a position to offer suppliers enough money up front to reopen and retool factories and to invest in safety measures, training, and hazard pay for the workers it would be asking to risk their own health? Chris was proposing to put Ventec at existential risk, on the assumption that a government contract would somehow materialize to help cover the cost—even though the federal government was already proving sluggish helping address simpler shortages for protective equipment and tests.

But, Chris figured, might as well try.

On a Saturday, March 14, Chris went public with his improbable vow that his little company was going to help rescue as many people as it could or break itself trying. He told *Forbes* magazine that Ventec could ramp up production fivefold within the next three or four months. He included a warning. "The time for action by the government is now," he said. Covid "is most likely to get worse by next fall."

■   ■   ■

That same night, March 14, an open letter started zooming around the Internet, its authors and signatories just as impatient to help the country deal with the pandemic, and just as unwilling to wait for the slumbering beast of the federal government to bestir itself in the country's service. Rachel Romer Carlson was in her early thirties, running a wildly successful education technology startup in Colorado. Kenneth Chenault, nearing 70, had been the CEO of American Express and had retired into Silicon Valley venture capital. The two of them put together a manifesto urging business leaders to help contain the virus and get resources to frontline workers, and started pushing the hashtag "#stopthespread." By the end of the weekend, they had more than a thousand signatures and a network of CEOs committed to pitch in and help, however they could.

Chris didn't know any of this until he got a LinkedIn message the following Tuesday, March 17, about a network of philanthropists ready to give Ventec money. He was on the phone with representatives from Carlson and Chenault's movement a few hours later. The group didn't yet have a name for itself—eventually it went with Stop the Spread—and was simply a collection of well-resourced people trying to do something about the virus. Two things really. One was to get certain in-person businesses—restaurants, bars, stores—to close to protect employees and customers, even where local governments hadn't yet asked. Two was, in the absence of any apparent coordinating authority in the public sector, to direct resources and expertise to meet need, particularly in getting supplies to hospitals, and capital to struggling small businesses.

Chris explained his own resource predicament. By now, in addition to the flood of orders for ventilators, Chris and others at Ventec were also fielding hundreds of phone calls from people offering help: neighbors hoping to volunteer in the factory or Google executives wondering how to be useful or wealthy individuals offering to just wire cash. One successful serial startup entrepreneur called to say he could send over $10 million right away, so that Ventec wouldn't have to wait on some cumbersome government procurement process to get the capital it needed. *Go buy parts!* was the message. *Go make ventilators! Go, go, go!*

Mere money wasn't going to cut it: There was nothing to spend it on. No one had yet been able to solve that fundamental problem. But it just so happened that Carlson's group had connections in auto manufacturing, an industry with vast global supply chains and manufacturing capabilities at mind-boggling scales. Within hours, Chris and some colleagues were on a follow-up call with two GM executives, trying to see what could be done.

It was a different kind of phone call than the others Chris had been taking recently, many of which involved well-intentioned people describing what they could do and asking to help. The GM execs instead began by asking what problems Ventec was trying to solve. Chris worked his way down his list. Supply-chain snarls that seemed impassable for a small-scale medical-device start-up turned out to be simple for a manufacturing mammoth with suppliers all over the globe. If GM couldn't find a part, the company could get it made, because it also had access to an industrial base that could put together metals and plastics. If a factory had shut down and sent its employees home, GM could provide the up-front capital and the safety protocols to get the doors open again. Plus, while Ventec didn't have enough workers or space, GM had plenty to spare after suspending production, furloughing thousands of employees, and leaving factories idle.

It all sounded promising, even if GM and Ventec were wildly

different companies with wildly different objectives, practices, and missions. Chris barely believed that a car company and a medical-device company could team up—they just didn't seem to match. Building cars must be complicated—Chris had no idea— but building ventilators was complicated in a different way. The machines had about 10 subassemblies, each of which needed to be checked with specialized testing equipment to calibrate and verify that it worked. The testing equipment itself had to be custom built. Would hospitals trust ventilators made by a car company?

Would they have a choice?

They didn't, probably, and neither did Chris.

The Paramedic

Road Trip

"Hey, I'm headed out to New York."

In tandem with its expected ventilator shortage, New York was also struggling to get people to hospitals in the first place, so overwhelmed were its emergency workers. Which was why Chris Cary got this bizarre phone call from his dad while at work, minding his own business and filling vending machines. It was March 26, a mild, cloudy Thursday in Colorado, the afternoon caught between predictions of wildfire risks and a possible snowstorm bearing down for the weekend. And here was his dad on the line, serenely announcing his plan to run straight into the flames of the pandemic. Chris spent about a second being surprised, and then he wasn't.

No matter that Paul Cary was in his sixties with a bad back and a blood clot disorder and who knew what other health problems generated by his decades of driving ambulances and refusing to rest. That was the kind of thing family and friends worried about, and Paul ignored. Paul was well aware of reports from the epicenter of the pandemic, at the other end of the country, of paramedics and hospitals besieged by the new virus—that was precisely why he was determined to go. Just the day before in New York City, health officials had reported 20,011 cases of Covid and 280 deaths from the disease; a doctor at the hard-hit public hospital in Elmhurst, Queens, had called the scene "apocalyptic." Colorado's governor, Jared Polis, had meanwhile issued a stay-at-home order, joining 20 other states, and pleaded with residents "to sacrifice to save the lives of our fellow Coloradans and our fellow Americans."

As an "essential worker," Paul had no plans to stay home and a much bigger sacrifice in mind. Colorado was experiencing no crisis comparable to New York's. The known death toll stood at 19. It seemed to Paul that the greatest need for his services, the chance to truly see and even slightly bend history, was elsewhere. This was not the first time he'd been seized with such a notion; he had volunteered to deploy to New York after the attacks of September 11, 2001, but never wound up getting the assignment. In the years afterward he often thought of the 343 firefighters killed trying to rescue people that day, and posted tributes to them on his Facebook page on 9/11 anniversaries.

Having been denied the chance to serve in that disaster, he now faced one that promised to be deadlier by orders of magnitude.

"Uh, okay," Chris said. (He decided against saying: *What the fuck, dad, are you serious? You know this is attacking old people, right?*) "When?"

"In three hours."

Of course. There wouldn't have been time to talk him out of it, anyway. This left, maybe, time enough to see him briefly on his way out of the state, to let him say goodbye to a grandkid or two among Chris's three sons. Paul no doubt would think Chris was being dramatic, but Chris knew just as well as Paul did what age range of people Covid preferred to kill.

Chris himself was 40 now, having grown up a fire department paramedic's son with all the attendant anxiety that entailed. As a kid, his younger brother Sean had sometimes cried himself to sleep worrying that his dad might run into a burning building and never come out alive. In reality, though, Paul's job involved more rescues than fires.

There were only three times Chris could remember that he didn't want his father to go to work. The first time he was probably seven or eight, and his dad, on the way out the door, said "See you next year." Chris was upset by this—why was his father disappearing for an entire year?—until he realized it was December 31, and his dad would be returning as usual at the end of his 24-hour shift.

The second time was when Paul was set to retire from the fire department before going to work full-time for a private ambulance company, and Chris kept thinking about a Denver firefighter who had died a mere 15 shifts shy of his own retirement a few years before, asphyxiated by smoke after running into a house fire. On Paul's last shift, Chris prayed his dad wouldn't have to respond to a fire—and of course his dad ended up having to respond to a fire. He got out fine. He had a retirement party.

This was the third time.

Chris got a few cases of water from work and insisted his dad stop by to get the bottles for the 28-hour drive across the country. He then went out to shoot hoops with his two younger sons,

Eli and Zach; the court was right off Interstate 70 on Paul's way out of town, an easy stop ahead of what promised to be a grueling road trip. The private ambulance company Paul worked for now, Ambulnz, was sending a dozen people in six ambulances to New York from Colorado, and expected them to get there by Saturday morning, so Paul and a partner were going to spend the night driving, taking shifts at the wheel. The plan was to spend a two-week deployment helping out New York's overburdened emergency workers, along with hundreds of other volunteers from around the country.

But first, Paul's company-issued blue ambulance pulled up to a high school basketball court, where Chris handed off the water, and Paul distributed hugs to his son and grandsons. Chris tried to push away a clutching sense of foreboding.

■   ■   ■

Paul had always wanted to be a fireman. His own dad had been a fireman in Denver, and when Paul was a teenager he would go stay in the firehouse and do whatever work the firemen didn't mind giving to a 16-year-old kid. He attended the fire school at Oklahoma State and got to live in a firehouse there, too. The Campus Fire Station had classrooms to train aspiring firefighters in flame-defeating techniques and breaking into burning buildings, and students helped pay for their room and board by going out to actually do the job.

Paul talked about firefighting all the time, including to a girl named Sue who he first met at a party and then shared a political science class with during freshman year. To Sue, he gave the

impression of being outdoorsy even though he wasn't, really—
being from Pennsylvania, she figured that he must, as a Colora-
dan, be into nature, plus he wore hiking boots, jeans, and a down
jacket, and sported a beard. He struck her as a kind person, too,
pretty quiet except for when he chattered about his work, and
once they started dating they'd hang out at the local burger joint
with the other kids from the firehouse. Paul earned his associate's
degree after three years, and the two got married and moved to
Colorado, where they stayed with Paul's parents till they found
an apartment.

Paul wound up with the Aurora Fire Department in the late
1970s, a few years before Sue gave birth to their first son, Chris. The
beard morphed into a mustache, a firehouse tradition with murky
origins; one popular theory suggested it came about because a wet-
ted mustache could filter smoky air in the days before breathing
aids came into use. (Also, unlike a beard, a mustache didn't inter-
fere with the seal on an oxygen mask.) The shifts were 24 hours on,
24 hours off, in a three-day cycle followed by a four-day weekend,
and though Fire Station 7 was a hectic one, based off a busy street
near the entrance to I-225, Paul found that fighting fires, by itself,
didn't seem to give him enough work. He soon started studying
to become an emergency medical technician (EMT), which meant
that in addition to his normal fire duties, he had to train for a certain number of hours in hospitals. He was working in a hospital,
in fact, the day his younger son Sean was born, even though Sue,
nine months pregnant, had asked him to try to avoid it. When her
water broke, she had to call the emergency room to try to hunt him
down. He did make it to her bedside in time to greet his new boy.

He got his EMT certification and then kept going, taking on more advanced training to become a paramedic. Whereas an EMT was authorized to perform a number of basic life-support functions—doing CPR, administering oxygen, setting fractures, treating burns—a paramedic could give the most advanced care available outside a hospital. A paramedic could do anything an EMT could do, plus run intravenous lines, administer a wider variety of medications, shock a patient's heart awake with a defibrillator, or even insert a breathing tube down a patient's throat. (Some paramedics joked that doctors had it easy—they got to intubate patients on adjustable beds with buttons on them and lamps nearby; a paramedic might get stuck doing that on a basement floor.)

Training on top of his existing job was demanding and stressful, but as the kids grew up, he still had time for school pickups, church on Sundays and Wednesdays, and Bible study. He'd show up to Chris or Sean's basketball games in the fire truck with his whole crew. The family knew ahead of time if he'd have to be on shift for a holiday or a birthday, and they built new traditions around that. Some Christmases he was gone, so they'd open presents on Christmas Eve. Some Christmas Eves he was gone, so the kids would each open a single present on Christmas Eve and take care of the rest when he returned from his shift on Christmas morning.

Still, being the family members of a firefighter, whose job it was to run toward disaster, meant that their home in Aurora held a kind of ambient worry. Paul had a fire radio at home that for a time remained on constantly, until one day when he was out during a major snowstorm and Sue could hear him telling colleagues over the airwaves that he'd gotten lost. He made it home eventually, but from that point on Sue kept the radio turned off. She didn't need the extra fear of being able to know everything that went wrong. As a kid, Sean knew that the firehouse chaplain and his dad's best friend from the fire academy were responsible for coming to the Cary house and informing the family if Paul died in the line of duty. His greatest worry growing up was they'd get that knock on the door, see the two of them, and know his dad was gone.

The risk was remote, however. Aurora's fire department had never lost a fireman. During the major fire Sean could remember from his childhood—a Village Inn experienced an electrical short that burned down the restaurant—Paul wasn't even on shift.

Paul was an affectionate if quiet dad who, when he wasn't home, made sure to phone his kids every night and answer their questions about what kinds of calls he'd gone on. The boys were in their church's equivalent of a Boy Scout troop, called the Royal Rangers, and Paul would help them make those little wooden race cars to send down a ramp. But work found a way to creep into those family moments. One year they built an ambulance, and another year a fire truck. Family road trips required stops at fire museums. Paul took the kids to a fire parade every year he was off for it, where antique fire trucks and rigs from different cities would go down the main street honking their horns and flashing their lights.

Eventually, after Paul got his paramedic certification, he felt an old restlessness resurfacing. Just as firefighting by itself hadn't been enough work, prompting Paul to do emergency medical training, he ultimately found that being a fire department paramedic wasn't really enough either. He had 10 days a month on a 24-hour shift with the fire department, and he sought more work elsewhere, picking up shifts driving ambulances for a private ambulance company on his days off.

The more time he spent away from his family, the more he was constructing another one for himself among the emergency-services crews and the doctors and nurses he saw in the hospitals he visited. If he was reserved and kept to himself at home, he came alive at work, freely distributing hugs and hellos among emergency-room staff and asking after their families, befriending everyone in the Aurora medical system, from the nighttime housekeepers to the trauma surgeons. A room full of overworked nurses and techs would light up when Paul came in, bringing with him his aura of calm and purpose and joy in his work. He would visit patients he'd brought in, because he just wanted to make sure everyone was okay, even strangers. Maybe especially strangers. He believed that love and laughter were "two of the best free medicines around."

In the world he lived in, he would go from eating dinner to becoming part of someone else's worst day. And then, at least when his children were younger, back to the firehouse to call home, to at least have his voice there while the kids were tucked in, even if in reality he was sitting on the bumper of a fire truck or washing blood off of his hands.

He also knew the job meant that you'd lose more than you won, but you still had to show up to play. He was known for keeping his cool, a reassuring presence to the younger EMTs and paramedics, fond of saying things like, "When you see me worry, then you can go ahead and worry."

His family continued to worry anyway. Sean harbored that fear of the knock on the door until the day his dad retired from the fire department.

When that day came in 2010, Paul didn't even want to retire. But things were changing, and he was changing, and the firehouse population was much younger than it used to be. He was in his fifties then, afflicted with a back ailment that had sent him into surgery on a Thanksgiving Day and rehab for months afterward. He still walked slowly. He didn't tell his family all the details, but they suspected he'd been strongly encouraged to move on, which he did by going full-time with the private ambulance company he'd been working for on his days off.

At home, meanwhile, the back surgery and the aftermath seemed only to have reinforced his reserve. Paul had always been quiet and rather serious but for the occasional dad joke. But now he drew further into himself. Paul and Sue had been accustomed to Monday breakfasts with one couple, bowling outings with another, but over time he lost interest in maintaining the friendships. When the kids had been younger they'd played every sport, sometimes two per season, and Sue had been too busy ferrying them from basketball to swimming to dwell much on Paul's absence. Now the kids were out of the house, and she and Paul were supposed to be retired, traveling, having fun. He simply did not want to stop working, though, despite the physical toll and his slowing pace. What looked to Sue like Paul's devotion to work over wife was becoming intolerable.

Sue didn't question Paul's fundamental kindness and compulsion for giving. The problem was, each person only has a finite amount of self to offer to the world, and the more one distributes it outside the home, the less one has to bring back. His focus was so trained on other people's crises that it sometimes felt as though he couldn't see the crisis gathering at home while his back was turned. His marriage was deteriorating, and he seemed to lack the will or the attention span to stop it.

After 37 years together, Paul and Sue divorced in 2012.

The months that followed brought a further cascade of personal tragedies for Paul. After the divorce, he moved in with Chris and Chris's wife and three sons, taking over the basement of their Aurora townhouse until he could find his own apartment in Denver. In the fall of that same year, Paul's brother, who had battled addictions for years, committed suicide. His mother died the following February, and his father in June.

Sue had remained close with his parents, and friendly with Paul. They sat together at the funerals.

Whatever the upheaval in his own world, there was a limitless supply of other people's worst days to show up for. To the extent that he'd long found in work a reprieve from whatever he wished to avoid in his non-work life, he was finding, with the loss of his marriage, his parents, and a sibling, less and less non-work life remaining. He put in years' worth of hundred-hour weeks—he wanted to be there all the time to help if he could, but sometimes he would get sick and even wind up in the hospital himself. At one point he developed sepsis, and had to have a medication-delivering catheter inserted into a vein and threaded all the way up near his heart, a device known as a peripherally inserted central catheter (PICC) line. He tried to go back to work with it still sticking out of his arm, but wasn't allowed.

■ ■ ■

That Thursday in March 2020, after leaving his son and grandsons, Paul and his partner drove all night, the highway cutting across Colorado's Eastern Plains and into the flat monotony of Kansas, then Missouri, Illinois, Indiana, Ohio. They took turns sleeping on the passenger side as the country slid past the windows and the states smeared together. They kept going until they hit Allentown, Pennsylvania, on Friday afternoon.

The directive relayed by Ambulnz had been to get to New York by 8:00 a.m. Saturday or risk being sent home. (Why New York would want to send anyone back when the city needed so much help was never made clear.) In addition to Paul's rig, the five other ambulances making the trek from Colorado—another from the Denver area and four from Colorado Springs—had pushed straight through as fast as they dared to drive, as no one wanted to schlep across the country only to get turned away. But as the fleet neared the city, the instructions changed, from "pedal to the metal" to "not so fast." So the Colorado crew of six EMTs and six paramedics ended up at a hotel in Allentown, just a few hours outside the city, where they actually got to sleep in a bed. New York was just about two hours away.

Paul was anxious to get to the city, to drive around and give what he could in his one little corner of the crisis. If ever there was a time he expected to lose more than he won, this was it. Just over the course of his roughly 27-hour road trip, 100 more people were reported dead from Covid in the state of New York, bringing the state's official death toll above 430, with most of the victims in New

York City. The United States had overtaken China as the global epicenter of the virus—at least according to official case counts, which you couldn't necessarily trust, in China because of officials' track record of concealing the extent of the virus's spread, and in the United States because there weren't enough tests to identify cases. Just two weeks before Paul's trip, not a single person was yet believed to have died of Covid in New York. The coronavirus was ripping through the state with astonishing speed.

Better to light one candle than to curse the darkness, even when the darkness was the most powerful Paul had yet seen in his decades as a paramedic. So many people were having their worst days now, including the overwhelmed paramedics of New York City. And here they were, marooned in Allentown as New York's 911 system risked drowning in a deluge of desperate phone calls, and people gasped for air—or endured more "ordinary" ailments such as gunshot wounds, broken bones, heart attacks—while waiting hours for ambulances to arrive.

There just weren't enough vehicles in New York to meet the demand to begin with, and the first responders were falling sick themselves. Some 200 had already tested positive for the virus. From a daily baseline of 4,000 medical calls, the 911 system took 5,700 calls on March 24, which two days later jumped to 6,000, and then 6,200 a day after that, smashing its own records multiple times in just a week.

Hanging back in Allentown, Paul was briefly suspended between home and Armageddon, right on the doorstep of a crisis with nothing to do. He at least recognized some of his comrades in medical arms. There were his Denver colleagues, of course. And one of the

Colorado Springs paramedics, a woman named Alissa he'd met a few months prior, when he'd driven the hour over from Denver to pick up a shift just because there was work available. He hadn't brought a partner—maybe no one had thought to assign him one, no one had thought to tell him to bring his own, or somebody he was supposed to work with had bailed on the shift at the last minute—and found out that he couldn't do a shift without one. It was Alissa who had greeted him and chatted with him briefly before he shrugged and drove the hour back home. Not long after that, Alissa had messaged him to get the phone number of a hospital in Denver where she had to transfer a patient who needed better care than what was available in Colorado Springs. He offered to take the patient there himself; she was touched, but said she really just needed the phone number.

The plan on March 27 in Allentown was to get some sleep, and then everyone would meet in the lobby at 7:00 a.m. the next day to head into the city. When morning came Paul was prompt and eager, and also irritated that a few stragglers didn't show up on time. He was the oldest in the crew but seemingly the most anxious to work. Finally, the caravan pulled onto the highway, and soon they were trundling across the Hudson and into New York City.

The Nurse

The Worst Shift

March 28–March 29, 2020

THE DAY PAUL CARY arrived in New York City on March 28, Michelle Gonzalez was working the worst shift of her seven-year career as a nurse. Thirty years old, short and loud with a brown ponytail and a Bronx swagger, Michelle cruised the hallways of the hospital with the self-assurance of a popular girl in high school, a backpack with a "Bernie" button slung over her shoulders. She was a nurses' union rep as well as a caregiver, and she'd lean in close to ask after colleagues' troubles with management, touching a companion's arm for concern or emphasis: "What's happening, ma? Tell me."

The problems she now faced, along with her colleagues, were on a completely different scale. No amount of fighting the power was going to fix them. The hospital where she worked, the Moses campus of Montefiore Medical Center, about five blocks from her home in the Bronx, didn't have enough of anything to fight the invisible monster preying on patients and caregivers alike.

They didn't have enough tests—Michelle was convinced that one particular patient who had arrived at her second-floor medical ICU about three weeks earlier around March 5, brain-dead from a mysterious cardiac event and suffering from two weeks' worth of fevers, had been among her first Covid patients. But no one had tested the woman because she was not expected to survive, and the hospital didn't have tests to spare.

They didn't have enough ventilators. Not two weeks after Michelle's encounter with that patient, a respiratory therapist had raced by Michelle wheeling a ventilator and asserted that it was the last one in the hospital. New York governor Andrew Cuomo had begged the federal government to send more ventilators to the state from the nation's emergency stockpile, and on March 24 had decried a promised shipment of 4,000 as coming nowhere close to matching the state's expected needs. "You pick the 26,000 people that are going to die," he'd snapped, addressing the federal government at a news conference.

They didn't have enough space—doctors and administrators were scrambling to find extra nooks to stuff patients into, lining them up in hallways, cramming extra rows of beds into the emergency room. Soon an old auditorium would be decked out with beds, too.

And they didn't have enough personal protective equipment—PPE, the formerly obscure acronym for the gowns, masks, face shields, and gloves that were becoming extremely scarce, except at the center of a national scandal: the richest country on Earth couldn't seem to find enough flimsy cloth and latex coverings to protect its medical workers. The *New York Post* splashed onto its front page a photo of nurses wearing Hefty garbage bags for gowns, accompanied by the headline "TREATED LIKE TRASH." Doctors and nurses started a viral hashtag campaign to "#GetMePPE"; Montefiore emergency-room staff started a GoFundMe drive to raise money for the materials, ultimately netting more than $60,000. Other scrappy operations were popping up: Cat Navarro, a suddenly out-of-work film-industry art director in Brooklyn, was marshaling a team of colleagues in movie props to source clear vinyl and glue-gun face-shields together; Rhonda Roland Shearer, a woman the media dubbed "the patron saint of PPE," was going hundreds of thousands of dollars into debt to find and donate supplies.

All the individual generosity and ingenuity was a response to a systemic failure no grassroots efforts could fix. The United States had not been prepared for the sudden spike in demand for protective equipment, and as governors pled for help getting supplies, the president at first dismissed them, declaring that the federal government was "not a shipping clerk" and leaving state officials to fend for themselves. Meanwhile, the federal government had ignored early warnings from officials to ramp up PPE manufacturing and was also perilously dependent on imports of protective equipment from China, which, facing its own shortages, was claiming domestic production for itself and buying up other scarce global supplies. A combination of long-standing manufacturing trends toward offshoring and short-term decisions to downplay the crisis had left America hopelessly behind, its governors trying to outbid each other in international markets for lifesaving equipment.

This meant that Michelle and her colleagues were reusing masks over and over, day after day, which prior to the pandemic would have gotten them disciplined for violating safety protocol. Nurses had to sit through mandatory classes every few years just to review how to safely put protective equipment on and take it off. (*Do not doff in the patient's room; use a separate doffing area. Do not touch the front of the gown. Shimmy out through the sleeves and roll the gown away from the body. Wash your hands. Remove the mask by the straps, away from your face, and discard.*) The risk of cross-contamination, infecting one patient with the disease of another, had been drilled into them so thoroughly that Michelle pronounced herself stupefied by this policy change in the midst of a highly infectious scourge. During the first week in March she'd been attending one of the routine "don and doff" classes, half paying attention to material she already knew cold, when she noticed something different. The instructor was telling her and her colleagues to remove their masks, place them in a plastic bag for later use, and then wash their hands again.

The practice was the hospital's effort to cope with the PPE scarcity even as its leaders tried to follow rapidly changing guidelines from the CDC. Montefiore was in no position to fix nationwide shortages of masks and other equipment, which left administrators to devise ways to protect staff and patients as best they could. But Michelle was appalled. Even the manufacturers' packaging on the now-scarce N95 surgical masks the hospital used—the good ones that filtered 95 percent of particles out of the air—displayed a crossed-out "2," as in, *do not reuse*. A friend of hers, another young ICU nurse named Taeler Danhieux, often said of PPE prior to the pandemic that you should pretend you had poop on your gloves so you would make sure they didn't touch your face, and she felt the same way about the outside of a used mask. The instruction to wash hands after removing the mask reflected that it was soiled. And you were supposed to put it in a bag and later put it right back on your face? Besides, Michelle wondered, wouldn't a plastic bag just incubate germs?

She was never satisfied with the hospital's answers to these questions, but at least there was ultimately a slight policy tweak. The masks were to be stored in paper bags instead.

Michelle and her colleagues found themselves going to more and more absurd lengths to conserve equipment and avoid infection, but there seemed no way to do both at once. She was being asked to take off her contaminated PPE inside patients' rooms—another departure from the old protocol—to avoid spreading infection in the hallways, at the risk of standing unprotected in the poisoned air. When this involved removing her mask, she was to hold her breath until she got out of the room.

Michelle managed to secure extra N95s for colleagues from donations to the nurses' union, but the shortage was unrelenting. She tried soaking a mask in an apple-cider disinfectant, supposedly a natural cleaning agent and safer than Lysol, only to find herself choking from the fumes when she put it back on her face. Colleagues who witnessed the resulting coughing fit stared at her in alarm.

"It's not Covid!" she gasped.

But other colleagues were starting to get sick.

One of the hospital's own nurses had wound up on a ventilator and under Michelle's care. The case followed an emerging pattern of severe Covid infections, in that it offered up cruel moments of false hope. On Thursday, March 26, the nurse-turned-patient had seemed to be improving enough to warrant removing the breathing tube, only to have it reinserted when her lungs couldn't function well enough on their own. It scared Michelle, seeing a sister nurse lying there, knowing it could be her or really any one of them. She was scared, too, on the next day, during the Friday afternoon when she and a respiratory therapist made plans to remove the tube once more; but if they had to insert it again a third time, they might have to make an incision in their patient's throat to do it. She just hoped the woman's increased steroid regimen had reduced the inflammation in her lungs enough so that she could breathe on her own.

Though Michelle was nervous for this second attempt to free her colleague from the fetters of her breathing machine, she was going to do whatever she could to wake this lady up. As she started reducing the patient's sedation, Michelle filled the room with her booming Bronx accent. "Hi there! How *are* you?! You okay?? Listen, today we're going to take the tube out, okay?? Can you wiggle your *finger*??" Michelle wiggled her own finger in front of the woman's face. She picked up her patient's legs, one by one, and pushed them around to try to help rebuild her motor skills. She put pennies on a table and instructed the woman to pick them up and put them in a cup. Michelle was trying to wake up the woman's brain, as the patient had been under sedation for perhaps two weeks. The grogginess she must be feeling now wouldn't be like coming out of a too-long nap; she would have woken up to a different world.

Michelle stood by as the respiratory therapist pulled the breathing tube out and gave the patient an oxygen mask. She was on guard for ICU delirium, a condition in which long-sedated patients become confused or even hallucinate and lose track of where they are. Michelle went through a series of questions to determine the patient's state of mind, starting with trying to reorient her. "Are we in the *supermarket*?" she trilled sweetly, as if teaching vocabulary to a small child. "Are we in the *library*?" Shakes of the head. "What *year* is it?" A puzzled expression. "Who's the *president*?"

Michelle could see the answer dawn on her patient slowly. "Oh," the woman croaked through damaged vocal chords. "That man. That, that stupid orange man."

Good enough. Her colleague was coherent and breathing. This was a source of hope for Michelle, if not quite optimism. The disease was astonishing in its destructiveness. But its victims could be astonishing in their resilience.

■   ■   ■

The next day was Saturday, March 28. Paul Cary was pulling into New York, and Michelle had put in a series of 12- to 13-hour days, had lost probably five pounds because she had had no time to eat, and was fighting symptoms of what she thought was exhaustion. She tried to ignore her mind as it wailed at her to slow down. Breathing was hard, and she alternately blamed her mask and her asthma. Her manager had told her that she shouldn't be so worried—she was only 30! Low-risk! But Michelle saw it differently; she was going home every night to a three-bedroom apartment she shared with her parents in their sixties and her 89-year-old grandmother with dementia. "Okay, so when I kill my grandma, is that going to be my fault?" she snapped. That ended the discussion.

Age was hardly perfect protection, anyway. She'd already cared for two patients who were the same age, both men, both 36. One made it, one didn't. It made no sense. No one had warned her that they were going to lose otherwise healthy people in their twenties and thirties.

Michelle had been caring for only Covid patients for weeks, and only the very sickest ones, who showed up in intensive care, breathing tubes and IV drips snaking into their bodies, unable to breathe on their own. The patient surge had come quickly—the Montefiore Health System estimated its case count had gone from two to nearly 700 in two weeks in the middle of March—and it had transformed the very landscape of the hospital. Hallways were lined with taped-up paper bags where the nurses stored their masks. Because medical workers were trying to reduce their exposure to their own patients, the floors outside patients' rooms were a thicket of tubing that ran from the veins of the person inside to IV pumps and medicine bags dangling from silver stands outside the door, so that nurses could monitor and swap out medications without having to step into a Covid room.

Overnight a seventh-floor unit that normally housed patients recovering from surgery had been turned, incompletely, into an intensive-care unit. That's where Michelle had been dispatched from her usual perch on the second floor, a proper ICU, with its line of desks facing patients visible through glass walls and its specialized equipment for critically ill patients. The new unit was a poor facsimile, and things started going awry soon after Michelle showed up at 7:00 a.m. on March 28 for her 12-hour shift. An intensive-care nurse should generally only be caring for two patients at a time, to allow for close monitoring and quick intervention if something goes wrong. That morning Michelle had already been assigned three patients, and she worried that each additional patient increased the risk for all of them. What if she was taking one patient's temperature and couldn't see that another was going into cardiac arrest? All of these people were so desperately sick, and now they might be in even greater danger because the hospital didn't have the staff to tend to them properly.

She pushed into her first patient's room, struggling against the door. Like everyone else, she was trying to limit how much time she spent in those rooms and how often she opened the doors to avoid letting the air spill out into the hallway; Covid patients were supposed to have negative-pressure rooms that pulled the air inside, to avoid precisely this problem, but the slapped-together ICU didn't have that, and the patients were coming in too fast to allow for retrofitting the building. She'd put on the full gamut of protective gear, the gloves and the face shield and everything else, before noticing that she'd forgotten to put on her N95 mask under the shield, and berated herself as she carefully removed the shield and fixed her mistake.

She had a protocol: The first thing was to take the patient's temperature. And the first thing she saw once she retrieved the thermometer from its bracket on the wall was the error code on its screen. "E3." Broken.

She swore and stalked back toward the door. She was already taking off her face shield and mask and holding her breath. She struggled with the door again; it was so heavy that she briefly thought she was locked in the room and might pass out from oxygen loss before she could escape. *They're going to find me on the fuckin' floor*, she thought. Finally she burst into the hall.

The rest of the shift didn't go any better. Electronic monitors inside the rooms failed to connect to the monitors at the nursing stations, as they were supposed to in an ICU, meaning that nurses couldn't monitor vital signs. If something was going wrong with a patient, someone would have to be physically in that patient's room to know it, and no one could be physically in all those patients' rooms at once. Another patient came in for Michelle, doubling her usual patient load; the person was massively overweight, and it took a serious effort involving several other people to wrestle the patient off the stretcher and into the hospital bed. A different patient's heart started beating irregularly, a potentially life-threatening condition called arrhythmia, and it took Michelle an hour to find the necessary equipment to administer the proper drugs.

She returned exhausted to the apartment she shared with her family. Here, too, she had started to observe a protocol, trying to keep them from getting sick. Michelle would call when she was a few minutes from home, and stand outside the door. Her mom would pass a plastic bag out and close the door again. Michelle would strip in the hallway, wedging herself into an alcove to try to hide, because the apartment was on the first floor opening out into the lobby. She'd spray her shoes with disinfectant and leave them in the hall. She'd empty her pockets, get out all her pens and her phone and ID. The clothes went in the bag and the other stuff had to be wiped down with disinfectant. She'd sanitize her hands before she walked in, still without clothing, and skitter right to the bathroom to take a shower.

The point of all this was to keep the disease out of the apart-ment. But Michelle suspected it had gotten in somehow anyway. Her dad was suffering from a fever, and her mom seemed to be coming down with something, too; she prayed they both just had colds. She felt guilty that she so often came home to describe her days of watching people die of a disease her parents themselves might have. But Michelle felt overtaxed by what she was seeing and by all the fear she felt for her own safety, and she needed to vent in order to keep herself from going crazy. With fury toward the bosses and administrators she felt weren't doing enough to protect the staff, she exploded to her parents: "They're trying to kill us!"

She'd been trying to convince herself she was fine, to avoid calling out sick. It was her job as a nurse to shove aside her own pain and fatigue and just keep pushing, and especially now, there was really no time to do otherwise. But she was horrified that this place that was supposed to help restore health was becoming an incubator for the very disease from which patients were trying to escape.

When Michelle finally collapsed into bed that night, sweats and body aches assaulted her dreams. When she woke up on Sunday morning she took her temperature. Her home thermometer, at least, worked. Her fever was 102.

■   ■   ■

New York City in March was the pandemic's American epicenter, and the Bronx—its poorest borough, home to around 1.4 million people—was the epicenter of the epicenter. There, the virus had inflicted its highest confirmed rates of infection, hospitalization, and death among all of New York City's five boroughs; once infected, according to one newspaper's analysis, a Bronx resident was almost three times as likely to die from the disease as someone in wealthier Manhattan. "Underlying conditions," those fearsome health factors that could determine whether the disease killed, brutalized, or barely touched a person, were legion in the Bronx: high blood pressure, diabetes, obesity. The South Bronx neighborhood of Mott Haven was nicknamed "Asthma Alley," the result of pollution spilling off the surrounding highways, and fumes from two sewage treatment plants close by. If you were to take the No. 4 train five stops, from Manhattan's East 86th Street on the Upper East Side to 138th Street in Mott Haven, the average life expectancy of those around you would drop by nearly a decade, from 86 years to 78.

Out of all 62 counties in New York State, the Bronx's ranking in health indicators, year after year, was 62nd, dead last.

More than 60 percent of Bronx residents were Black or Hispanic, and the borough's own underlying conditions helped to explain why, across the country, such communities were getting hit the hardest by the disease. These included poverty, lack of access to health care, and crowded housing. Social distancing might be impossible in a 44-story public housing project with unreliable elevators, and quarantining wasn't an option in a one-bedroom apartment shared by a mom, a grandma, and six kids.

Nor could many people work remotely. The Bronx was where many of New York's "essential workers" lived, the nurses such as Michelle, the transit operators such as her dad, the grocery clerks and security guards and garbage truck drivers. While much of the city tried to shut down and stay home, commutes into and out of one Bronx neighborhood actually increased as its residents kept parts of the city running for the day, if it ever came, when New York would resume its hyperactive rhythms. Rich New Yorkers could flee to the Hamptons or Cape Cod or anywhere else in the country with a little more space. The essential workers of the Bronx needed to stay put and keep showing up. And then they'd go home, often out of sight of their richer neighbors who relied on them.

Michelle had spent her whole life in the Bronx, a place she loved and mourned for at the same time. For much of her childhood, she had shared a one-bedroom apartment with her parents, two siblings, and grandmother, so that when the family finally moved to a three-bedroom the same year she became a nurse at 23, Michelle thought it was basically the Taj Mahal.

It was still the hood, as she described it with defiant pride. Growing up there had meant growing up without heat and hot water, being advised by her parents to get under a car to protect herself if she heard shots. It meant her high school didn't have mats for her cheerleading team to fall on doing stunts; they'd have to stay up or hit the hard floor, a harsh but effective incentive to avoid mistakes. (She only found out that other teams had mats when she attended competitions at other schools. *So this is how white people live!*) It meant going through a metal detector when she got to school.

It also meant a community of working-class people enduring the crime and the general difficulty of living, just trying to get by. She'd watched her parents do it: raise a family and do a decent job at it in cramped quarters. Her dad Ernesto, whose friends called him Papo, worked a subway booth. Her mom Carmen worked at the post office until carpal tunnel forced her retirement, in addition to caring for her own mom and a brother with cerebral palsy.

Michelle gave them both credit for that now. It was a harder thing to do here than on the other side of the class divide, in the suburbs of Westchester or New Jersey, where people had sweeping lawns and sent their kids to good public schools. It wasn't until Michelle went to college, a few neighborhoods over from home in the Riverdale section of the Bronx, that she even realized what she was missing. She'd visit friends' houses in the suburbs and find herself ogling the trees, amazed by the fact of roses in gardens and people living in so much space, with heat, not realizing their neighbors, in the hood just down the road, didn't have that—not thinking about people like Michelle at all.

For a time, those people, what they had that she lacked, were all Michelle could think about. But if Michelle's upbringing had deprived her of many material comforts, it had also provided her with her life's purpose. She learned from an early age how to be a caregiver: Her uncle Peter's cerebral palsy had held him captive in a wheelchair for life and inflicted on him a variety of other health problems. Michelle had learned, for Peter's sake, how to use a nebulizer to administer a mist of medicine to his lungs, and how to operate a Hoyer lift to get him out of bed and into his wheelchair. She helped to cook for and feed him on the weekends, though she wasn't above whining to her mother about the high school parties she missed while she did all this. But she also realized she was growing to like the work, and that she could offer care for other people's families, too.

Montefiore Moses was the neighborhood medical center, about five blocks away and up the hill from the new apartment. A brick building a block wide anchored the complex, its green angled roofs giving it more the bearing of a high school—one of the nice ones— than a hospital. It was one of 15 hospitals in the Montefiore Health System, distributed through the Bronx, neighboring Westchester, and further upstate, an empire that had sprawled up and out from its modest origins as a "home for chronic invalids" founded on Manhattan's Upper East Side in 1884. Michelle knew it well from frequent visits with Uncle Peter.

She also knew about the institution's problems. Even in 1884, the original institution had faced overcrowding, with more applicants than available space; by 2018, an irate Bronx city councilman, Ritchie Torres, was condemning an "epidemic of hallway placements" with patients, particularly poor ones, being left on cots jammed into hallways. One such patient, 87-year-old Louis Collazuol, complained to the *New York Daily News* he'd had to put a blanket over his head in order to get any sleep because the hallway lights never went off; he figured that anyone walking by his bed would think he was dead.

Michelle's mom eventually got so fed up with the way Peter was being cared for at their neighborhood hospital—it was always too busy, and he sometimes waited hours for treatment, sitting in the emergency room with other sick people—that she started taking him to a different hospital a 15-minute drive away. Michelle thought Peter wasn't getting the respect or attention he deserved as a patient because of his disability, which also made it impossible for him to stick up for himself.

"That's kind of why I'm a fierce advocate for fighting for people," she explained. She got into union work, haggling with management for better contract terms for her colleagues, pushing for better staffing, and decrying overcrowding. "People who don't have voices—I'm gonna have a voice for you. Because I got a big mouth."

She didn't expect that she'd wind up fighting her own hospital for the sake of her parents. Or that she wouldn't win.

The Chef

Shutdown

NIKKIA RHODES WAS a fighter too. She had to be. She was 23 years old, a restaurant chef and a schoolteacher, a biracial woman in the South whom a white relative had referred to as "nigger," declaring her name to be too "ghetto." Her father had been in and out of prison for much of her childhood while her mother struggled with drug and alcohol addiction. Meanwhile, her city of Louisville, Kentucky, in the pandemic year of 2020, was not only wracked with disease and economic devastation, like so many other cities around the country and the world, but would also become a focal point in a fight over race and policing that engulfed the United States over the summer, after a cop killed an aspiring nurse named Breonna Taylor in her home—and that movement would sweep up Nikkia and give her a mission to feed and heal her community.

But Nikkia was still teaching culinary arts to the public school kids of Iroquois High, and Breonna Taylor was still pulling emergency-room shifts as a technician, in March when the pandemic first found its way into Kentucky. Covid took its time ambling around the state as it lay waste to lives and livelihoods elsewhere; while case counts exploded into the thousands in New York in the middle of the month, Kentucky's were still hanging out in the dozens.

The state did however have a few canaries in the economic coal mine heralding the disaster to come. Louisville's biggest employer, accounting for 20,000 of its jobs, was United Parcel Service (UPS), and the company's air hub in the city was running daily flights to China before the pandemic hit. In late February, UPS started to warn of declining demand and supply-chain disruptions. And Kentucky, its economy dependent in part on tourism related to horse racing and bourbon, was poised for particular hurt as travel and gatherings were discouraged to slow the spread of infection. The Kentucky Derby alone brought $400 million annually to Louisville, and already in February, officials were fretting that the May event might not go on.

Meanwhile, face masks were disappearing from local stores before the virus was even detected in the state—despite the CDC's guidance then, later reversed, that members of the general public didn't need to wear them—and grocery chains were imposing caps on purchases of hand sanitizer and certain medications.

Yet when the inevitable happened, and Kentucky reported its first Covid case on March 6, the governor reassured the state that "Kentuckians remain at low risk."

Iroquois High stayed open, and Nikkia kept pushing through a school year she'd begun with a lot of hope that by now was submerged in frustration. This was her second year teaching at Iroquois, the first of which she'd spent using PowerPoint to try to teach kids how to cook, as the school didn't even have a kitchen or a budget for ingredients. Iroquois served a poor community not three miles from the sweeping lawns and graceful columns of Churchill Downs, home of the derby and mecca of thoroughbred horse racing. Just down the road from all that opulent wealth, some 80 percent of Iroquois students were poor enough to qualify for free lunches, and the school catered to a large refugee population in the surrounding neighborhood, including kids from Somalia, Congo, and Iraq. The math and reading scores were perpetually dismal, as was the graduation rate. A town where the horses were better cared-for than many children: That was the unequal Louisville Nikkia knew.

The first time she'd walked into her classroom in 2018 she seriously questioned her decision to take the job. The carpet was moldy, the ceiling tiles were rotting out, and Nikkia's mandate would be to keep 150 kids, from freshmen to seniors, occupied for the year, somehow teaching a culinary class without any actual food.

She taught lessons on food safety and sanitation, and brought in as many guest speakers as she could—an official from the health department to explain how restaurant food grades worked; a fire department sergeant to discuss fire safety (if grease ignites in the kitchen, *do not* throw water on it); an employee from Little Caesar's to demonstrate how to fill out a job application, because many of her students would have to start working right away.

The school had promised to build her a kitchen for the 2019–2020 school year, and she'd looked forward to seeing the kids do the kinds of things that had meant so much to her when she'd taken culinary classes at their age: working with their hands, making food

they'd never heard of before such as Hollandaise sauce. But circumstances mocked her optimism, and as fall swept a new school year
into session in 2019, Iroquois kept finding itself in the local news—
the principal was assaulted; some kids got into a major, bloody fight
in the bathroom; other kids set off fireworks inside, which everyone
thought were gunshots.

On March 9, Nikkia was sitting through a teachers' training,
annoyed that she wasn't in her own classroom with her own students. She had to go to these sessions periodically because, in the
five years since she herself had graduated high school, she'd worked
in restaurants and hadn't trained in education. The program also
catered to retirees who had spent, say, 20 years in plumbing, and
now wanted to educate others, and Nikkia's own proximity to her
high school years was exactly what made the classes so tedious for
her. She hadn't spent decades on another career, and she knew
pretty well what high school teaching was supposed to look like,
and not look like, from the chalkboard-facing seats. One of the reasons she'd wanted to do culinary education in the first place was
that, as much as she had loved her own classes, she was convinced
she could do them better than her teacher had.

She passed some time scrolling furtively through her phone,
something she might have scolded her own students for, reading
about this new virus infecting people overseas. Some were saying
it was a kind of flu; different countries were reacting in different
ways. And then, as she sat there, she saw a news article reporting
that Italy—the whole thing—was shutting down.

An entire country has shut down. What's about to go on? she
thought. *Never heard that in my lifetime.*

The next day she checked in with her aunt, who had respiratory problems and was closely monitoring news of the virus. Western Kentucky University, Nikkia's aunt informed her, was already closing, planning to bar students coming back from spring break.

Nikkia knew, once that happened, that her high school would be among the next to close. Back in the classroom later that week, her students kept asking questions about the virus. But this wasn't like demonstrating the difference between a chop and a dice and a mince, and Nikkia couldn't guide them. She didn't know herself what was going to happen. On Friday the 13th, only half the class came to school.

In the early hours of that same day, Breonna Taylor died on the floor of her hallway, bleeding from multiple gunshot wounds. Local news outlets at first reported an unidentified woman's death in an "officer-involved shooting"—one of two such deadly incidents to occur that same day—the full details of which would not become clear until weeks later. For Nikkia, the early reports barely stood out from the pattern of violence in her community, where the murder rate was rising, as was the number of police shootings, with mostly Black suspects getting shot. Besides, there was this virus to worry about.

On Monday, her school shut down.

■   ■   ■

The school's shutdown was only supposed to last a few weeks, till April 6. And as the weeks unspooled, the costs mounted. Congregating was now considered dangerous. Preventing "community spread" meant community was collateral damage, and entire people-facing industries such as bars and restaurants closed up shop to visitors, with a stroke of the governor's pen, the same day Iroquois shuttered itself. Not only were kids out of school, but more and more Louisvillians were out of work—especially lower-income Louisvillians who relied on service jobs. Nikkia's mother, Dawn, who had worked her way up at a Logan's restaurant from making $2.13 an hour plus tips as a server to $12 an hour doing food prep, got laid off herself.

Around the country, according to one survey, some two-thirds of restaurant workers had lost their livelihoods by the end of April. The millions of such jobs that had evaporated amounted to a fourth of total job losses across the United States that month. An industry that had nurtured Nikkia's young career, that had helped her celebrate special occasions or soothe bad days with meals, and for which she had been preparing her students, seemed to be disappearing before her eyes.

As Nikkia confronted how in the world to teach culinary classes remotely—especially to a set of students who didn't necessarily have their own laptops or WiFi connections, who might be trying to care for siblings or sick relatives, whose parents might have lost their own jobs—she knew from her own difficult childhood exactly what they stood to lose. Not just a classroom, but a refuge. And not just training, but a purpose.

Both school and restaurants had saved her, and not so long ago. Just six years before, they had set her on a path to teach and try to guide the kids who might be struggling as she had.

As a kid, Nikkia had only a fragmentary understanding of why her dad was mostly gone, incarcerated for drug possession or the robberies he undertook to pay for his addictions. From behind bars he would draw pictures he'd send home for her to color in. Once, he sent a poster-sized drawing of a teddy bear with hearts bubbling into the background. He'd doodle cartoon puppies and monkeys on the envelopes of the letters he sent her. He also stole from her. During one of his last stretches of freedom, when Nikkia was in high school, she and her mother returned home from an outing on a Saturday morning to find Nikkia's Nintendo Wii gone, along with the DVD player. Dawn knew right away who was responsible. "This," she told her daughter, "was your dad."

Dawn sought a restraining order. The court date happened to fall on February 19, Nikkia's birthday, where she beheld the shattering sight of her father, a Black man with a strong build from having worked out all the time in prison, looking weak, in a wheelchair, his skin an ashen gray. He'd been suffering from colon cancer.

He apologized when she visited him in the hospital the next day; he called her up to apologize again a day or two later, saying he'd gotten her some candy for Valentine's Day and her birthday, but had eaten some of it himself because his blood sugar was low. She told him it was fine. She felt at peace with him.

He died a few days later. Nikkia was 17.

Around that time, she and her mother were living with Nikkia's godmother. Nikkia hated being there; her godmother would get angry at her for not doing the dishes and take her mother's food-stamp card to shop for herself. Yet when Nikkia was hungry, she would generally find in the cabinets years-old canned goods well past their expiration dates. She came to dread eating at home and found herself more and more absorbed by her school's culinary

program, where she could feed herself and vouch for the ingredients. Schoolwork and food: These were things she could control, in which set steps yielded predictable outcomes and regular
rewards. There was psychological and physical safety to be found in
the halls and classrooms of Louisville's Western High. She studied
hard. She got good grades. She got elected class president going
into her senior year.

She picked up a restaurant job, too, at a trendy place called
Milkwood that advertised its fare this way: "Southern Inspiration
+ Asian Flavors + Bourbon Cocktails." Her first few days happened
to coincide with derby weekend, a time of profitable chaos for the
city's restaurants, so she kept her head down and her hands moving, hurrying salads and appetizers out of the kitchen. That job led
her to a training and apprenticeship program run by Milkwood's
owner, Chef Edward Lee, that aimed to put youth from underserved neighborhoods on a pathway to employment in a growing industry. Through Lee's Youth Hospitality Program, Nikkia
learned food prep and office management and menu planning, and
threw pop-up dinners with classmates. Years later, she could still
recite the menus from memory: succotash with velvety corn puree;
okra; cream puffs filled with Benedictine spread, that creamy
cucumber preparation people spread on crustless sandwiches for
the derby. She was especially proud of one dessert, a cobbler pop
tart, peaches and simple syrup in puffed pastry, topped with a basil
ice cream.

As she learned the food industry, she kept searching for ways to
be the kind of person she wished she'd had growing up—a stabiliz-
ing force and a navigator to a better life. She thought she'd found

it at Iroquois. But now she couldn't offer the sense of safety she'd discovered at school to other young people, facing who knew what problems at home.

Her students missed three weeks of school entirely while administrators scrambled to set up technology for remote schooling and provide computers and Internet access to the kids who didn't have them. The district superintendent pushed back the reopening date to April 20, then May 1. Teachers received no particular schedule to follow for virtual classes, but were simply encouraged to get their kids to learn somehow. Borrowing an idea from a colleague, Nikkia put together a chart of activities her students could complete for points, with 10 points a week required: Read an article on family food traditions and send in a family recipe; make a new recipe with a family member and send in photos or a TikTok video of the process; clean out the pantry, get rid of expired food, and try to donate still-good food you won't use. She concentrated on trying to help them cultivate skills she knew they'd need no matter what the world became. They'd have to eat, and hopefully they could feed others, too. She felt lucky to be teaching a subject that students could stitch into their everyday lives.

But as remote learning wore on, she was also watching kids she'd never seen struggle in person start to fall behind online and take hits to their GPAs, mere high schoolers being forced to navigate new adult struggles. A parent out of work might be unable to pay the Internet bill, so the student couldn't even attend classes. Or the parents still worked outside the home and the older kids needed to watch their siblings. Nikkia knew of students who didn't have enough to eat at home, or whose caretakers died of Covid and who suddenly had to figure out how they were going to fend for themselves and their siblings. By the start of June, researchers were already warning that educational disparities between racial and socioeconomic groups were set to get worse outside the classroom. Nikkia's students were in exactly the groups poised to lose the most.

The hoped-for May 1 reopening came and went and the school stayed closed, all the way up through the tail end of May, when her students got to mark getting through the virtual slog with yet more screen time and distance from friends. Graduation was on video; seniors got signs to put up, in yards or in windows, in silent recognition of their achievements. The school district was doing its best, running bus ads listing the names of graduating seniors, lighting up stadiums, getting graduation speeches aired on local radio, but Nikkia ached for those kids because they wouldn't get to experience what she had. Some of her seniors would be the first in their families to graduate high school, but would mark the moment the same way they had spent the last months of their senior year: isolated and on a computer. Just a few years before, Nikkia's own graduation, as class president, with her name the first to be called and her speech about greatness (or something, she couldn't quite remember) propelling her peers into the lives that awaited them, or maybe just forcing them to sit through one more thing before the whole experience could be over with—that graduation was a big deal for her family. Her mother hadn't graduated high school, her brother hadn't graduated high school, her dad was dead, and still there she was. It was not a ticket out of a difficult life by any means, but it was proof that triumph was real, that sometimes, even in hard times, you did, in fact, win.

She knew students whose immigrant families had been waiting for this moment, for the chance to see their first generation become *American* high school graduates, for their kids to claim a piece of the country's much-vaunted opportunity. Now they were graduating with both their celebrations and their prospects cruelly kneecapped, into a horrific recession featuring nearly Great Depression–level unemployment, with an estimated 20 million Americans out of work by May. Even though Covid overwhelmingly spared children and teenagers from its worst physical effects, it had utterly warped the world around them.

Nikkia wasn't worried about her students' GPAs. She was just hoping they survived this new world.

■   ■   ■

Breonna Taylor's story showed that survival wasn't something to be taken for granted. By the end of the school year in May, Nikkia had seen Breonna's biography take shape over social media and in news reports, as family and friends filled out details of her life and the circumstances of her death. Just like Nikkia, Breonna had attended Western High School, graduating a few years before her. The teachers there spoke highly of Breonna, and Nikkia believed them. The school's youth service center coordinator, Stephanie Holton, told a local Fox affiliate that Breonna was the kind of student who might find another girl crying in the bathroom and bring her to Holton for help. "She looked out for the students other students didn't look out for," Holton said.

Breonna had wanted to become a nurse, perhaps in neonatal care, because, as her mother later told a reporter, she liked babies but not kids. She had once worked as an EMT, but at the time the pandemic hit, she was serving in two different emergency rooms as a technician. Her mother worried for her safety at work and kept urging her to wash her hands. Breonna was reportedly unfazed, responding that she had to do what she could to help. She was essential, after all.

But just about a week after the virus officially showed up in Breonna's state, on Friday, March 13—her night off after a series of 12-hour ER shifts that week—police showed up at Breonna's door. First they knocked, then they used a battering ram to break the door down, later saying they did so after hearing no response from inside. Breonna's boyfriend said later that he fired a warning shot at the floor, not realizing the intruders were police, wounding one; officers unleashed a salvo of retaliatory fire, killing Breonna.

Breonna's wasn't the first killing of an unarmed Black person in 2020 and wouldn't be the last. Her death followed that of Ahmaud Arbery, 25, shot as he jogged near his Georgia home on February 23, and preceded that of George Floyd, 46, whose killing was caught on camera when a Minneapolis policeman knelt on his neck for more than eight minutes on May 25.

Nikkia couldn't watch the video herself. Her family had its own experience with the police. In brief periods of her childhood when her father wasn't incarcerated, he would sometimes come home with a busted lip and explain that he'd been tackled by police. When she looked at George Floyd, she saw her father.

Millions of people did watch the video, which stood as a horrifying indictment of police brutality, with its searing image of a calm white police officer casually pushing his knee into a Black man's neck, hands in his pockets, while his victim begged for help. It caught fire across the country in a way Breonna's death hadn't at first, drowned out as hers was early on by a cascade of pandemic news. But just because America was grappling with a new crisis of disease didn't mean it had shed its old ones of racial strife and violent injustice. Suddenly Breonna's name was being chanted alongside George Floyd's as protesters marched demanding justice, first in a handful of cities and then in many more. Louisvillians were among the first to rally in solidarity with protesters in Minneapolis and in recognition of their own pain.

Nikkia marched among them on May 26. She joined nervously. She feared the virus as well as the police, either of which she thought might kill her. She determined to mask up and stay distant from other people as she marched, because she knew she couldn't bear to sit out the protests, and she told herself she'd rather die fighting for justice and equality than hide from Covid.

A few days later, Nikkia got a call from one of her friends in the restaurant business, Lindsey Ofcacek, checking on how she was doing with everything going on. "With everything going on"—that was what people said now, a blanket reference to pandemic, police brutality, protests, any other curses 2020 cared to mete out. Lindsey worked with Nikkia's old chef mentor, Edward Lee, and had cofounded with him the restaurant-employment nonprofit Nikkia had worked with in its early form. Now called the LEE Initiative (for Let's Empower Employment), at Lindsey's behest the organization was busy helping to feed thousands of food workers who had lost jobs overnight when restaurants shut down en masse. Through the Restaurant Workers' Relief Program, closed restaurants in 19

cities had already transformed themselves into relief centers, offering food and supplies to the struggling.

That was a national project for a national problem. But Lindsey
could see that Louisville's pain after Breonna Taylor's death, and
then George Floyd's, was bigger than job losses. Violence clearly
threatened people's lives, but so did lack of basic access to food,
and both of these scourges disproportionately menaced Louisville's
largely Black neighborhoods. This had been true even before the
pandemic, but the disease laid bare so much hurt and so much need
that it was hard to know where to even begin to help. Lindsey told
Nikkia that she didn't do well just sitting in the chaos, not being
able to be part of the solution.

Nikkia understood, and thought she heard in Lindsey's voice
the mind-set of a white woman trying to help heal. Nikkia's own
mind-set, though, was that of a biracial woman just trying to hold
it together for friends and family. She wanted a way to get involved,
but was struggling with her own pain, too, and just didn't know
what else to do.

But then Lindsey hit on an instinct the two of them shared:
feeding people. The prep kitchens of shuttered restaurants across
the city were lying fallow while people went hungry. And Louisvillians had lost a source of comfort and community at a time when
comfort and community were precisely what they needed. What if,
Lindsey suggested, they started up a community kitchen?

Nikkia figured they could end neither the pandemic nor racism. But they could cook. And the more they discussed it, the more
Nikkia saw a purpose take shape for her as a chef and an educa-
tor. School was out; Nikkia's students could help staff the kitchen,

where they'd learn culinary skills as well as a sense of service. She wanted them to have a positive and safe outlet to participate in the city's racial justice movement, without running into the police's rubber bullets. "Some people," she told Lindsey, "feel called to march. Others show up in different ways."

The two of them dug straight into logistics. How many meals did they want to serve? What kind and where? They agreed they wanted to feed entire families and to offer hot meals—not sandwiches and chips and pasta salad, but a big tray of something home cooked that a family could take home and pop in the oven. Nikkia had no problem with cold lunches but felt that a hot meal showed just a little more effort, and a little more caring.

They hung up with plans to meet soon and hash out more details. But before they could do that, more protests would convulse the city with the release of new details about how exactly Breonna Taylor had died.

Louisville and the nation had already lived through months of disease, isolation, economic deprivation, and uncertainty. The U.S. Covid death toll stood at nearly 100,000 on May 25, the day George Floyd died. Yet it was still very early in America's dark hour, and before the summer was out, the country would endure a summer surge of virus infections as well as a wave of protests and racial anguish. People who had been avoiding crowds or stuck for weeks under stay-at-home orders were pouring into the streets, as politicians and public-health officials fretted the protests could spread the virus further. Millions of protesters in thousands of cities and towns across the country opted to take their chances and demonstrate over the summer, generating, in the midst of a pandemic, what was possibly the largest movement in United States history. Mayors vowed reforms; police chiefs stepped down; George Floyd's killer was arrested and charged; Breonna Taylor's was fired three months after shooting her. Where protests were accompanied by riots and vandalism, individuals and businesses already hit with pandemic losses sustained $1 billion to $2 billion in damage across 20 U.S. states.

And before Nikkia and Lindsey could settle on what exactly they wanted to do to help, another shooting would tear a new gash into their wounded community.

PART TWO

The Patient

Downhill

March 20–March 27, 2020

H<small>UY'S MOM DETERIORATED</small>. The doctors kept giving her more oxygen, but it didn't seem to be helping much—not enough of it was actually getting through her inflamed lungs and into her blood where it belonged. She had already spent days in the hospital, with Huy's sister calling in frequently to check on test results and prognosis. By Monday, March 23, her fourth day in the hospital, one of Liên's doctors was recommending intubation, while another kept advocating to avoid the ventilator and pump up the oxygen support. The disease was too new, and doctors were only now learning how to treat it, with people like Liên serving as involuntary educators. She was confused and frustrated.

One point of consensus, however, was that the infected had to suffer more or less alone—or rather, in the company of strangers, medical professionals who risked infection themselves to be there. She couldn't have her family beside her to help her decide what to do. Instead, they gathered virtually at her bedside on Face-

Time. There Huy saw his mom, who had survived a war and a dangerous sea journey from her home, who had started a new life in America, and put her husband through school, and had run a store, and raised a family, lying there weak and disheveled with all these tubes sticking out of her.

Huy didn't know why, but he hit record on the conversation. Maybe it was a premonition of something bad to come. Maybe it was just to preserve that moment of the four of them together.

He was worried, helpless to fix anything. And his mom, with her family forbidden from visiting her, was facing the terrible choice of whether to outsource her own breathing to a machine. Huy was an engineer; he knew machines failed all the time. Should his mom really entrust her life to one? On the other hand, would she survive without it?

It was too much; Huy started to cry. All the news coming out about this virus was bad. California officials were worried about running out of bed space in hospitals. Stanford University had already shut down its campus for the rest of the academic year. This rich land his parents had come to fleeing communism was now, incredibly, facing toilet-paper shortages.

For her part, Huy's mom seemed more irritated than anything else. She was annoyed that the doctors seemed not to know what they were doing with this disease, whose behavior was still a virulent mystery, with no cure or even reliable treatments. Liên was out of patience and incredulous that medical professionals couldn't seem to get their shit together, and Huy felt a flicker of relief to see that his mom's sickness hadn't defeated her feistiness. But Huy's sister reasoned that if a doctor was encouraging

Liên to go on a ventilator, then it was probably the right thing to do. So it was settled: Liên would consent to the intubation, and her family reassured her that she would probably just be on the machine for a few days, that she just needed a little help breathing as she fought the disease. They'd see her when she woke up. And then she'd go home.

Huy didn't learn, until he did some research later, what his mom was about to go through.

She would have a tube, about a foot long and the width of a Sharpie, stuck down her throat. Conscious people tend to fight this process instinctively, and for that reason, once doctors decided Liên couldn't breathe on her own, there was a very important first step before the tube could go in.

Liên would be sedated and paralyzed.

At which point she really wouldn't be able to breathe on her own.

So the doctors would need to get her hooked up to the machine quickly. They would do this by inserting a metal paddle, called a blade but not actually sharp, into her mouth to move her jaw and tongue out of the way and get a good look at her throat. For some patients, in rare instances, this step could come at the expense of breaking a few teeth. But it was important, because the throat contains the entrances to both the windpipe and the esophagus (which is why things can "go down the wrong tube" and a person might have a coughing fit from accidentally inhaling a sip of water rather than swallowing it). If the ventilator tube went into Liên's esophagus by mistake, the machine would pump oxygen into her stomach instead of her lungs, and then she'd likely throw up and choke.

Meanwhile the person inserting the tube would have to get

very close to Liên's open mouth, a risky thing to do with a Covid patient. If she coughed, the virus could spray throughout the room and infect anyone who wasn't wearing the proper protection. Some medical personnel used intubation boxes, clear plastic crates placed over a patient's head with holes for an intubator's hands, to try to keep droplets or aerosol contained.

All this should only take 10 to 15 seconds, and the procedure was simple relative to what came next. Once the tube was in, the real battle began. A ventilator's settings control variables including oxygen saturation, the number of breaths a patient takes per minute, the pressure with which air is pushed into the lungs. Any one of these settings could hurt Liên if calibrated incorrectly. The pressure could be too high and pop a lung. The oxygen could be too low and fail to nourish the blood. Independent of any settings, the breathing tube could escort other pathogens into her lungs and cause infection. The very machine that might save Liên's life also seemed to multiply her risks.

■   ■   ■

Within days of checking his mother into the hospital, Huy found his own condition getting worse. On Wednesday night, March 25, two days after his mother's intubation, his lungs wouldn't let him sleep. He would start to drift off and then wake up fighting for air. Every time he opened his eyes, he would check the clock and find that barely any time had passed. The hours crawled by in this way. At some point he pulled himself from his bed and over to the couch, where he realized he could breathe if he was sitting straight up. He managed to sleep a few hours before daylight.

When nighttime returned on Thursday, he was set up on the couch with his blanket and pillows, expecting to pass the hours upright as he had the night before. He sat there watching television, trying to stay calm, trying to keep his breathing going. He liked the show *Naked and Afraid*, a survivalist reality program in which two stars, one woman and one man, get dropped into the wilderness without food, water, or clothing, and are filmed trying to make their way out. Sure, he was sick, but things could always be worse.

At his sister's recommendation, he was also monitoring his blood oxygen through an oximeter clipped to his finger. She'd explained to him that normally the meter should give a reading close to 100 percent oxygen saturation. "If it drops into the low 90s," she'd said, "that's concerning. If it drops below 90, get your ass to the ER."

Huy now watched that number drop. Mid-90s. *Just close your eyes*, he told himself. Low 90s. *Take deep breaths.* He tried to will more oxygen into his bloodstream, as if his brain could somehow do what his lungs wouldn't. *Everything's going to be okay.*

He glanced at the oximeter again. 88. Dread closed its fingers around his struggling windpipe. He knew he belonged in the emergency room.

But he was alone. His father had started to feel better and was out picking up medication. Huy called him. "I need to get to the hospital, now. You have to come and get me." Nghê rushed home; Huy could hear his father calling him from the door but found himself empty of the energy he'd need to respond. He could barely speak, much less make his way out of the house. His dad had to physically guide him off the couch and march him to the car for the trek to Stanford Hospital, where Facebook had referred him for his earlier Covid test. He'd been told then to come back if his symptoms got worse, which they had, precipitously. He'd be admitted about 15 miles northwest of the place where his mother lay struggling in her own hospital bed.

Before that could happen, though, Huy faced a battery of inquiries at the hospital doors. Nurses in full protective gear were manning the entrance and they were, as in Santa Clara, reluctant to allow anyone into the building for fear of contagion. They wanted to know if he'd been tested. Yes, he said, and it was negative, but he obviously couldn't breathe very well and the rest of his family was sick. A nurse told him that if the test was negative he didn't have Covid and should go home. Huy barely had the breath to argue but he knew he needed help. Finally another woman stepped out to inquire what the problem was.

"I got tested a few days ago," Huy pleaded, gasping. "It came back negative. My doctor told me to come to the ER if things got worse. Things got worse. They're really bad. I can't breathe. I don't know what to do." He explained his plummeting blood oxygen saturation.

At that point the woman rushed him inside, demanding oxygen.

Huy sat in the emergency room with an oxygen mask strapped to his face for about an hour before he was formally admitted and brought to a hospital room upstairs: fluorescent lights, white floors, machines beeping. He lay in a bed as people stuck things to him, another oximeter for his fingertip, electrodes on his chest, a tube called a cannula to feed oxygen into his nostrils. Every piece of missing protective equipment in the country seemed to have wound up at Stanford. Huy could barely recognize human beings under all the gowns and face shields and masks and bonnets. They were more like sci-fi creatures, slapdash robots scrounged from spare parts.

They ran tests; they confirmed that he was in fact positive for Covid. Wires stuck out of him and sensors stuck to him, tracking his oxygen and heart rates as they teetered just on the edge of dangerous. Turning over or sitting up could tip either indicator into unsafe territory and send a machine into anxious beeping. Not that there was any escape from beeping; this mechanical chorus was destined to become the soundtrack to his attempts to sleep. Which, somehow, he finally managed to do.

He woke with a screaming thirst around 8:00 a.m., but his nurses said they had to run more tests and couldn't give him anything to drink. Carefully, surreptitiously, he maneuvered a thermos of water out of his backpack, which now lay next to him on the bed, trying to sneak enough sips to soothe his throat without setting off extra beeps. Hours went by this way, with Huy growing steadily angrier, until he at last demanded that someone, anyone, just tell him what really was going on and why a hospital would deny him something as basic as hydration. A doctor arrived at his bedside to explain. It wasn't really about any tests. The doctor thought Huy would probably have to be intubated, and if he had food or liquid in his system he might choke.

Huy was livid. "I'm not getting intubated," he said. "This is fucking bullshit. I got admitted last night. And it's been however many hours and you won't even give me any fucking water?"

Eventually his doctors relented, but said they'd keep monitoring him to see if intubation was necessary. In the meantime, though, he was allowed to have lunch. Chicken noodle soup, some juice, as much water as they could bring him—because Huy feared they might not be bringing him water again.

After he ate, Huy lay still. He had the television on but his eyes were fixed to the oximeter, which kept teetering around the edge of 90, and any time it fell below, the monitor would start its maniacal beeping. He kept trying to lie back, close his eyes, and focus on getting enough oxygen. Doctors came and went, periodically suggesting that Huy should be moved to the intensive-care unit and put on a ventilator, and Huy fought it every time. "I'm not going on a ventilator," he insisted. "I'm staying right here." A nurse reassured him: "Everything will be fine. They can't take you anywhere against your will." She said she'd make sure of that.

Hospital staff sought other options. Someone brought Huy an inhaler and urged him to take a deep breath with it. This threw him into such a severe coughing fit that he couldn't stop for close to half an hour.

Not long after that, the nurse who was Huy's ally in his fight against going to the ICU showed up again with his doctors. This time she didn't comfort him. She just stood in the corner and looked at the floor.

"What's going on?" Huy demanded. She didn't say anything for a moment, as her companions started to grab Huy's stuff and prepared to wheel his bed into the ICU.

Finally, she murmured, "I'm so sorry."

The doctors explained that even if Huy didn't want to be intubated, he would be better off in intensive care—he'd get his own nurse instead of sharing one with five or so other patients on his floor. He could get more attention and be monitored more closely, and, given the state of his breathing, the doctors wanted to be able to respond to him quickly if needed.

Only days ago, he'd reassured his mother as she considered ventilation that she would make it out all right in a few days at most. But he knew now that she hadn't made it out in a few days; Liên was still unconscious with a machine breathing for her. He also knew the chances were increasing that he was about to go through the same ordeal. In which case he'd be unconscious and entirely indifferent to whether he had his own personal nurse.

But he relented. The doctors seemed determined, and he didn't have the energy to argue anymore.

The first thing Huy noticed about the ICU was how cold it was. Or maybe how cold *he* was; he couldn't tell whether the chill was a condition of the air or of himself. His new room was significantly bigger, so much so that he couldn't understand why he had all this space. A giant window faced onto the hallway, so he could see all the doctors, and they could see him.

He also learned very quickly that his fear of the ICU had been well-founded. Evening was approaching now, on the back of all the hours he'd killed begging for water and fighting transfer to the place where he'd ended up anyway. He wasn't there an hour before a doctor approached him to recommend again, strongly, that he be intubated.

Huy's resistance was weakening as the doctors kept pushing. This was why he'd wanted to avoid the ICU, but now here he was, having removed one last barrier between himself and the tube. He didn't like taking medication in general, and avoided it unless absolutely necessary. The thought of getting all those crazy drugs pumped into him to the point where he couldn't move or breathe on his own, and depending on a machine for his very life, with absolutely no margin for error . . .

He called his sister to ask what he should do.

"Don't make me make this decision," she told him. It had been she who had advised their mother to get intubated, and Uyên still wasn't sure she'd made the right call. "I can give you all the facts," she said. "But you have to make it for yourself."

Huy read off his vital signs to his sister from the screen by his bed: his heartbeat, his oxygen level, his respiration rate. She told him he was breathing at three times the rate he should be. An adult at rest should normally be breathing somewhere between 12 and 16 breaths per minute. Huy was taking closer to 40 breaths a minute. "You might feel okay now, because there's pure oxygen being blown into you," she said. "But you're breathing really fast and it's really hard to maintain those oxygen levels. If you keep breathing like this, your heart could give out."

Maybe he was hyperventilating because of the anxiety of hospitalization and everything else befalling his family, his sister reasoned, and maybe anti-anxiety medication would calm that down. But again, this was more medication, and there was no guarantee it would work, and in the meantime how much longer could his heart withstand all of this gasping?

Huy got off the phone and called a doctor back in. He wanted to know whether anyone else was on a ventilator in that hospital, and what their chances were. She wouldn't tell him no matter how he pressed—patient confidentiality. All she would say was that there were indeed other patients on ventilators in the same building at that moment, and things seemed to be going okay so far.

Just okay.

Of course it was his choice, the doctor said, it was just that the respiratory team qualified to perform intubations was leaving for the night within the next hour, and there was no guarantee a ventilator or even a bed would be available if Huy needed one tomorrow. Plus, if Huy did have a heart attack overnight, he would need an emergency intubation anyway. If he was going to wind up a knocked-out part-robot regardless, he might as well do it before the heart attack.

He was afraid. *What happens if shit goes wrong?* Shit, on the other hand, was going very wrong already. *What else can I do right now?*

One hour. That was the time Huy had to make a decision that might save or kill him. Death seemed to beckon from either side.

■   ■   ■

He was alone when he made up his mind. The doctor had stepped out into the hallway while he tried to consult with his sister and his father. He was exhausted, tired of fighting, and felt that if they had to do the intubation thing they might as well do it now.

He started waving at the glass, trying to get the attention of the doctors visible in the hallway. Now that he was resigned to getting on a ventilator, he wanted it over with, and he couldn't seem to get anyone who'd been so eager to intubate him earlier to come into the room and do it already. Finally someone noticed him, and he watched as everyone put all their gear back on to come in and learn about his decision.

Stanford had all the money in the world, it seemed, and did not appear to Huy to be suffering from any of the equipment shortages he'd heard were prevalent elsewhere. What they didn't have, Huy was amazed to learn, was a fucking clipboard. Huy sat on his bed paging through a floppy sheaf of papers and its thicket of legalese and liability absolution and do-not-resuscitates, and he absorbed the indignity of not really being able to sign it properly, the absurdity and the gravity all tangled up in a single moment.

In his haste to get through the documents, he didn't notice that he also signed up for a study for an experimental therapeutic drug, remdesivir, offering his body as a testing ground for a medication that researchers hoped could aid other severely ill Covid patients.

He spent a last few moments paying bills on his phone. Who knew how long he was going to be out, if not forever. Certainly he feared death, but there didn't seem to be much he could do about that now. More immediately, he feared late fees or a hit to his credit score if he was unconscious too long to take care of his expenses. Here was a problem he could solve, something he had some control over even as chaos crept in around him.

He tried to reassure himself, texted his dad and his sister to say they'd all get ice cream when he and his mom were both better. A nurse glanced at his chart and noticed that his birthday would be coming up in a few days, on March 31, and he believed her when she said, kindly, that the team there would do everything they could to make sure he didn't miss it. Maybe he'd be awake in two or three days to find his mom awake too, the whole family restored to health, and all of this would be a grim anecdote. A team of doctors introduced themselves to him and quickly got to debating what drugs to use and why the drip feed wasn't dripping.

Finally, one of them told him to start counting backwards from 10. *10, 9, 8* . . .

Then darkness.

The CEO

Down to Kokomo

H<small>UY HAD TRIED DESPERATELY</small> to avoid the ventilator, but nearly a thousand miles away, Chris was just as desperate to make sure patients like him could get one. Outside Seattle on March 17, he was on the phone with GM executives, daring to hope he was close to solving his problems. Ventec had already fielded plenty of offers of help that went nowhere or missed the company's real needs. The NASA Jet Propulsion Laboratory—literal rocket scientists!—had volunteered their services at one point but couldn't come up with anything Ventec actually needed. (Scientists there ultimately designed their own ventilator, a feat one of the engineers described to a Ventec executive as "really fucking hard.")

Meanwhile, Chris worried about being able to make any ventilators *at all*, let alone scaling up massively, because pandemic-driven factory closures and spiking demand were snapping the world's supply chains. Ventec got most of its parts in the United States, which was now difficult enough, but Chris was fixated on finding one piece in particular: the blower motor that actually moved air through the machine. Without this, there could be no ventilators, and everybody might as well just go home.

It so happened that this component was manufactured by a factory in India, and it also happened that said factory sat in a state that had shut its factories down. Prying open the blower-motor plant wasn't just a matter of strong-arming a vendor: It meant negotiating with a foreign government to jettison its own pandemic-safety measures just as its country's case counts were starting to spike.

So, Chris asked the GM executives, can we get that factory open? Their astonishing response: Yes, we can.

GM, unlike Ventec, had its own employees in India, and almost immediately dispatched people to the factory site itself to discuss what it would take to restart. Separately, Ventec and GM both worked State Department contacts to try to get Indian officials to allow the facility to operate. Within days the factory was functioning again, and GM workers were there helping it scale up.

That was one problem solved: Ventec was at least back in a position to make machines that blew air. All it had to do now was something it currently had no capacity to do: Make many thousands of them. Quickly.

■   ■   ■

More than decade earlier, Dave Good had been Ventec's second employee, when the company was two guys working out of an aircraft hangar. Once Chris decided to forge ahead with GM after March 17, Dave was one of his first phone calls. Formerly the company's vice president of manufacturing, Dave was now pushing 70 and retired, living in a fancy building in Portland with his wife and near his daughter and granddaughter, and had spent a pleasant few months getting to love the city's restaurants before all of them shut down. He was a thick-necked slow talker, with the bearing of a grizzled Vietnam veteran minus the actual grizzle, insofar as he was completely bald.

Chris needed to bring him out of retirement.

Dave, locked down in his penthouse, wasn't difficult to persuade, though he was just as skeptical as everyone else that GM could help make ventilators—maybe even more so since he knew the manufacturing process so intimately. But within days he was in a GM corporate jet with a few other colleagues on a mission to scope out factory space, a man well aware of his years and putting himself into an enclosed space with several people for hours while all around the country an airborne virus cut down people his age. He thought back to boarding the plane to go to Vietnam. That, of course, had been no corporate jet, but the feeling he had now was similar. He didn't know if he'd ever come back. *Man, I don't know,* he thought. *But it needs to be done, so here I go.*

The jet landed in a place called Kokomo.

This, as Dave could easily see, was not the beachy paradise off the Florida Keys that the Beach Boys had made up. There was no such place anywhere near South Florida. Instead there was an old Indiana manufacturing town flanked by cornfields, which dubbed itself the "City of Firsts"—home of America's first commercially produced gas-powered car, first stainless steel, first aerial bomb with fins, first canned tomato juice, mechanical corn picker, and transistor radio. The town was also, according to a roadside sign greeting entrants from the south, the hometown of Norman Ray Bridwell, author of the *Clifford the Big Red Dog* children's books, Kokomo High School Class of 1945.

It was GM territory, site of millions of square feet of factory and office space now idle in the pandemic. But it wasn't just fear of contagion that had hollowed out GM's sprawling complex of buildings and parking lots. In fact, GM had been whittling down its workforce in the town for years prior to the pandemic. Kokomo's economy had been socked by the decline of the auto industry and then the economic crisis of 2008 and 2009, and in 2008 had made a *Forbes* list of America's top 10 fastest-dying towns. The city's GM facilities had employed thousands of people, then only about 180, and then in 2020 furloughed the remainder to try to contain the virus.

Dave wasn't impressed as he toured through various buildings with a few GM counterparts. A circuit-board manufacturing plant was too full of walls and partitions. Other buildings looked more or less like warehouse spaces, and each one seemed dirtier than the last. One building, apparently the site of a past chemical leak, had a sign on the door warning against occupancy for more than 12 hours. He did not think it a promising location for the manufacture of life-support ventilators.

Finally, he pointed to a facility the group had not yet entered. "What about that one?"

"That's an office building," one of his GM counterparts said. "We can't manufacture in that."

"Well, let's just go look at it."

What Dave saw inside was a vast former office space, an abandoned cubicle farm that looked like it hadn't been used or updated since the 1990s. One could almost picture old "Dilbert" comic strips pinned to the fabric of the divider walls or the "World's Best Boss" and "I Hate Mondays" coffee mugs leaving dark rings on the desktops. In no way did it resemble a manufacturing floor, because it wasn't one.

Dave thought it was perfect.

The moment was like a movie scene in which the newlyweds walk into their dream house for the first time and *just know*. But instead of the charming colonial on a cul-de-sac with a fireplace and lots of closet space, this place had removable floors and movable desks and could become wide-open space. All it needed was a total transformation—cubicles out, ventilator factory floor in, along with complicated copper piping to get oxygen to the machines and make sure they worked. In Bothell, Washington, it had taken five months to put together the proper setup in a space about a tenth of the size.

Dave went back the next morning to take another look at the building and make sure he'd made the right call. The parking lot was no longer the desert he'd seen the day before; now it was filled with maybe 30 cars and trucks. Workers had been there all night taking office furniture, and seemingly everything else that wasn't nailed down, out of the building.

If Ventec was working with people like this, Dave thought, the insane thing they were attempting might actually be possible.

■　■　■

Chris arrived soon afterward around March 30, late at night, in a small prop plane that skidded to a stop at the Kokomo Municipal Airport, a tiny facility originally built as an emergency base for the military during World War II. He'd come with his best friend and co-conspirator, Chris Brooks, Ventec's chief strategy officer and a fellow alum of George Washington University, as well as a few other colleagues. All of them were goofy with fatigue when they climbed out into the chilly dark, feeling the depth of the obligation they'd taken on along with disbelief they were really doing this. They'd rented a GMC sport-utility vehicle to stay on-brand with their newfound manufacturing friends. The darkness was so powerful that Chris Brooks nearly drove the car into the grass before he found his way out of the airport and steered south into town.

As they passed the "Welcome to Kokomo" sign by the side of the road, Chris Kiple pulled up The Beach Boys song on his phone, and the carful of tired friends sang together woozily about getting away from it all and taking it slow, as they sped toward a once-abandoned building now being gutted at breakneck speed.

General Motors, having told employees to avoid work for their own safety, shifted gears to recruit people who would come anyway. The company's call for paid volunteers yielded an outpouring of more than 1,000 applications, and by the end of March 100 volunteer employees were taking safety training, five people at a time, on keeping apart and cleaning workstations. (This was also right around the time the president accused GM in a tweet of moving too slowly and invoked the Defense Production Act, more than a week after the Ventec partnership launched.) The factory was still under construction but would ultimately feature squirtable jugs of hand sanitizer at the entrance, temperature checks, and mandatory mask and goggle protocols for the factory floor, plus workstations spread six feet apart.

The Chrises arrived at the GM building around 1:00 a.m. Hundreds of people were there, some of them building up the factory space even as others started to make ventilators in it, with Ventec employees from Bothell instructing their new GM colleagues on the delicate art of building breathing machines, and auto workers from several different states rapidly learning an entirely new job in the middle of the night. GM's forsaken office building was alive with activity, transforming into a larger replica of Ventec's factory back in Bothell, complete with its subassembly testing stations and its bright white and blue walls and its silver wire racks. The first machines were scheduled to start rolling off the line within hours.

Emotion seized Chris Kiple, and his eyes fogged over. Now wouldn't be the time to deliver a pep talk about the historic nature of what everyone here was doing, how they were stepping up to a generational challenge and destined to save lives. Every single minute was vital, and a 15-minute rah-rah session for a few hundred people would be a lot of time lost. Still, he was looking at something far beyond the least-practical dreams in his head, hundreds of people working so hard and accomplishing so much in such a short period of time. He'd had no idea what people could do in the face of a crisis.

But this was only early spring, and the crisis was just beginning.

■   ■   ■

A few hours' drive from Kokomo, at a small community hospital on the north side of Chicago that Chris had never heard of, Dr. Suzanne

Pham was worrying about ventilators. She'd spent months bracing for the inevitable invasion, observing from news reports around the world how quickly Covid patients deteriorated from walking through a hospital's doors, upright and independent, to lying in a hospital bed, unconscious and helpless even to breathe on their own. The hospital where she'd worked for about a decade, Weiss Memorial, ordinarily didn't have a huge need for ventilator support, and the 19 machines it had were normally plenty to cover the hospital's small ICU with some left over. But Weiss stood surrounded by nursing homes and served mostly elderly patients, and once Suzanne saw news of America's first known outbreak at the Kirkland Life Care Center outside Seattle, she knew it was only a matter of time before Covid came for her neighbors, maybe for her, too. And she feared 19 ventilators wouldn't be anywhere near enough.

Few understood, when people first started getting sick at the Kirkland nursing home in mid-February, that they were dealing with a virus so deadly it would kill dozens of residents in the space of a few weeks. How could they know? It made no sense: No one there had recently been to China, and the handful of confirmed Covid cases in the country at the time nearly all involved people who had traveled to the center of the original outbreak in Wuhan or had contact with someone who had. The federal government was restricting tests only to those with China travel history or known exposure to an infected person, with the result that even if someone at the Life Care Center had suspected the real culprit, they wouldn't even have been able to check right away. None of the gasping, wheezing residents qualified for a swab for crucial weeks while the virus spread through the facility. It wasn't until February 29 that state officials confirmed the presence of Covid there, and then the chaos only mounted. Ambulances crowded the parking lot; medical workers, ominous and ghostly in their protective costumes, came and went, hauling out stretchers with patients who were ill, frightened, and confused. Family members with relatives inside stood at windows and tried to offer love and strength through glass; Life Care staff said they did all they could, always expecting federal help that did not come.

By March 18, 34 people were dead in Kirkland, and the moment Suzanne had been fearing arrived: Covid hit a nursing home in a nearby suburb of Chicago. Twenty-two infections became 46 in the space of a day. The state health department, which had already restricted visitors to long-term care facilities, now urged nursing homes to ban nearly all guests and social activities. Residents could no longer share meals together in the dining rooms. At the stricken Chateau Nursing and Rehabilitation Center in DuPage County, Illinois, moms and sisters, uncles and grandpas, cousins and friends were trapped and isolated in a sealed-up pen of cream-colored brick with infections coursing through it. This outbreak would be only the first of many in the state: Illinois nursing homes had up to 80,000 people in their care, and they also, a *Chicago Tribune* investigation found, had racked up more infection-control rule violations prior to the pandemic than did homes in nearly any other state.

But Suzanne knew that even measures that would ordinarily help protect residents from illness—regular hand-washing, food safety, and so on—couldn't necessarily stop the coronavirus from spreading once it struck inside a nursing home. Had it become sentient and gone into architecture, the virus itself couldn't have designed a better place in which to spread and kill, with dozens or hundreds of people, having the fragile immune systems of the elderly and in varying degrees of health, all living in close proximity; staff members going from room to room bathing, changing, or otherwise touching and breathing on people; visitors coming and going. Even though state officials had condemned so many seniors to untold loneliness in the name of safety, the homes' infections were destined to multiply.

The residents themselves, Suzanne understood, were practically defenseless on their own; other people's decisions would determine their fates. She had trained in pediatrics but, during her years of working with elderly patients at Weiss, had observed how life's beginning rhymed with its end, how both the very old and the very young depended so much on others for help and care. She believed the nursing homes near Weiss would try their best to protect their residents, and still she knew that many would likely die.

As case counts exploded within the nursing homes around Weiss, Suzanne was trying desperately to coordinate her own hospital's defenses, working with other physicians there to forge protection and treatment protocols out of ever-shifting guidelines from the CDC, state, and county health officials. She and her colleagues had begun in late February to test patients coming in with respiratory symptoms, but getting results always took days—days during which they had to find room in the hospital to isolate those patients, treating them as Covid-positive without really knowing what was wrong with them or the best way to help them.

So when Suzanne admitted the hospital's first official Covid-positive patient on March 23, she couldn't confirm the diagnosis until days later. But she was sure enough what she was dealing with that, after spending the day swaddled in protective gear and caring for her patient, she didn't know whether she should go home to her husband and two young children. She knew she needed them, needed their love and support and some sense of steadiness for what she was facing and about to face, and she knew the heart-sickening truth that for all her precautions, she might be exposed to the virus, and her very presence could hurt them. She went back to her family, hoping that the virus wouldn't chase her home.

After that first patient, the levee broke. In a matter of weeks, half the patients at the hospital had Covid; in a few more, the whole place was a Covid ward. As a young physician, Suzanne had been trained in how to deliver bad news to families, how to cope with death and dying. But nothing had prepared her for death on the scale she and her hospital saw now. Weiss was small enough that a Code Blue, indicating a patient's heart or breathing had stopped, was rare in normal times. Now she was hearing them multiple times every hour. A doctor could no sooner race to a coding patient's bed-side to try to stabilize that individual than another patient would go into cardiac arrest.

Weiss's ventilator supply dwindled. Suzanne was having discussions she'd never wanted to have as a doctor, conferring with hospital ethicists about how to decide who would get a machine and who wouldn't on the day they finally ran out. These decisions, if necessary, would likely be made according to who had the best chance of surviving. And she, along with colleagues, was calling around to other area hospitals, nursing homes, and manufacturers to try to get more machines. But so was everybody else, and the calls always seemed to go the same way. Other hospitals worried about running out themselves; ventilator companies were flooded with calls and swamped with back orders. The hospital's respiratory-care supervisor kept careful track of how many machines were in use, how many were left, and what other methods of ventilation the hospital had to provide support.

As March slipped into April and Weiss's Covid patient numbers kept rising, its number of available ventilators kept falling. Suzanne and her colleagues were searching everywhere for more ventilators, and no one could help. And then, finally, they found some hope. They found Chris Kiple.

■   ■   ■

In Kokomo, the scramble was on. Ventec and GM personnel converged on Kokomo from different parts of the country. Shuttered or sluggish local hotels flung their doors back open to accommodate the influx of trainers and engineers and construction teams and executives. Chris moved into a Hampton Inn and felt like he was back in college at GW, except with everyone in masks; people were working at strange hours of the day, coming and going, leaving their doors open, getting two hours of sleep a night.

It felt as though everyone was on their team. The mayor of Kokomo stayed up late getting permits ready for the factory. The guy who had designed the Corvette chassis for GM came through with a new roller-stand design. Once, Chris, wearing a fleece vest from Ventec into a gas-station convenience store in a vain attempt to get coffee, got stuck in a conversation with a cashier behind Plexiglass who was more stoked about ventilators than any cashier

Chris had ever encountered. Chris had been awake all night and really just wanted caffeine but had found the store's coffee stand emptied out because of Covid. He was too tired to engage much or to absorb the fact that he'd just been recognized at a gas station for the first time in his life.

Kokomo, clearly, was a welcoming place—notwithstanding local legend that the town's nineteenth-century founder, David Foster, had named it after an Indian chief he'd called "the orneriest Indian on earth" because "it turned out to be the orneriest town on earth." But Chris, subsisting on takeout and working constantly, barely had time to mingle. Every day brought new opportunities for the whole enterprise to go off the rails. Getting enough parts quickly remained a constant struggle. The blower-motor factory in India could only make so many items in a day, and GM was pushing for more. The factory resisted launching a night shift; its workforce was mainly made up of women, and they didn't want to risk walking home in the dark. Ultimately Ventec and GM bought hotel rooms for all the workers at the Indian factory to keep it running around the clock.

Other parts would get stuck in customs or move too slowly because of their labels—relevant officials couldn't tell from GM tags that they were dealing with medical-device components, and so didn't think to prioritize them properly. Meanwhile, the threat of infection loomed over everything. GM had shut down its factories early on for a reason, and whatever the Kokomo factory's mitigation measures, the Covid risk was real. Outbreaks would become a regular problem, necessitating quarantines along the affected production line and efforts to make up for the lost time in other shifts.

Still, just about a month after Chris's first phone call with GM executives, the partnership they'd forged was scheduled to ship its first breathing machines.

■   ■   ■

Chris Kiple didn't know until a few hours ahead of time where the new ventilators would end up. He spent much of the day on April 16 scurrying through the factory with Chris Brooks, tracking sub-assemblies as they came together and making sure each component passed inspection. Everything had to work for the first time, from testing the air compressors down to packing up the boxes and making sure they had the right accessories and shipping paperwork.

All the while Chris Kiple was on the phone with FEMA and the White House to figure out where the machines were even supposed to go. The first destination was to be a FEMA staging area at an airport outside Chicago for distribution to hospitals with the greatest need around the country. But it turned out that some of the most desperate hospitals were already quite close to home. Two more stops were added to the delivery tour: a hospital called Franciscan Health in Olympia Fields, Illinois, and Weiss Memorial, in Chicago.

At Weiss, Suzanne Pham wasn't sure exactly how her hospital had ended up on the short list to get new ventilators. She knew that White House officials had been calling around to hospitals to assess their needs, and that Weiss had been among them and developed a connection to the West Wing. She also knew that by the time a UPS trailer lumbered into the hospital parking lot on April 17, with a sign affixed to its back declaring "America, We Are Here With You, We Are Here For You," Weiss was nearly at a breaking point.

Watching the truck arrive, masked up and standing in the parking lot with several of her colleagues on that cool and cloudy day, Suzanne started to cry with relief. The machines had come with absolutely no time to spare; some of them would need to be in use on patients that same night. Suzanne had not only been caring for patients herself and coordinating the hospital's overall response; she and some colleagues were also working with nursing homes in their area to try to limit infections among their patients, to prevent as many as they could from winding up in the hospital in the first place. In the nationwide frenzy over PPE, hospitals got priority allocation of scarce supplies; some nursing homes near Weiss couldn't even get gloves. Suzanne and others at Weiss had worked the phones, helping their neighbors find suppliers and sharing safety protocols as health-care professionals learned more about the disease. She was seeing her community and her hospital come together—nurses in their sixties and seventies coming out of retirement to care for patients despite being at high risk themselves; hospital physical therapists, lacking patients to tend because they were all too sick, emptying trash and cleaning out rooms just to help.

Suzanne and everyone around her burst into applause as the UPS driver hoisted up the truck's sliding door and pulled out the cardboard boxes, scrawled with messages from Kokomo in multicolored markers. "We're all in this together!!!" "GMCH Kokomo Strong! #builtwithlove." "Keep on caring, we are with you." "God speed." A woman cut through the packing tape and Suzanne held up a device, to further applause. "These are lives saved, absolutely," she said. "Thank you."

Chris had arrived in Chicago himself mere minutes before a scheduled press conference to mark the feat he was still astounded they'd pulled off. His life over the past few weeks had become a series of minor miracles averting near-meltdown, so it was only appropriate that the Kokomo–Chicago commute had been the same, dealing him a flat tire en route as well as two Guatemalan Good Samaritans who pulled over to help fix it. Thus was he roughly on time to watch the first shipment of GM–Ventec ventilators come off the truck. This was a moment they'd all been working toward, and he knew that countless more such moments would be necessary.

Yet it felt wrong to celebrate. He had noticed the outdoor freezer in the parking lot, where bodies were being moved to because the hospital morgue was too full. Here he was, delivering a very small piece of the puzzle of trying to save lives, and struck with reverence for the health-care workers putting in 20-hour shifts at the hospital, fearing the day they'd have to ration ventilators, while Covid killed people around them.

He stepped up to a podium to deliver remarks in front of a banner thanking the hospital's staff—"Our heroes work here." The body deliveries to the outdoor morgue stopped for the time it took to film him, the hospital's overflow Covid dead relegated out of the shot and lurking just offscreen. "Something that we never thought would have been possible months ago, has been achieved," Chris marveled. About 5,000 people had been involved in getting these ventilators assembled and out the door in such a short period, at a time of such tremendous need.

He knew the magnitude of the triumph was relative: One giant leap for Ventec and GM, and one small step to meet the crisis still running relentlessly ahead of them.

The cameras switched off. The bodies rolled out.

The Vaccine Developer

Racing Ahead

February 6–May 15, 2020

Hamilton was making giant leaps of her own that, if successful, would eventually make most of those new ventilators unnecessary. The work was important and fulfilling, and the pace was punishing: In trying to launch the Moderna vaccine's first human trials so quickly, she was compressing into a matter of weeks a process that, at the record-setting speed of her previous Zika research, had taken up most of a year. She was a scientist, so she knew it was nonsense, but it did feel sometimes like the universe was trying to break her. When her Subaru stuttered to a stubborn stop on yet another late-night commute from the office on February 6, forcing her to get an Uber home, she collapsed just inside her front door and broke down herself, yielding to frustrated tears as well as the reality that she probably needed a new car. She couldn't work this hard and then have her car break down at 10 o'clock at night in the middle of Cambridge. She knew she was not mentally strong enough for that.

She selected another Subaru. She wouldn't get to use it much before the state shut down.

In the meantime, she spent her days coordinating among dozens of people on different teams within the company and potential collaborators outside of it. Every day she assisted the manufacturing team to try to find ways to make the product faster. She hunted for partners and funders. She contributed to research white papers. She prepared long-term development plans. She helped get paperwork ready so Moderna could ask the FDA to let the company start giving the vaccine to humans in clinical trials.

The vaccine manufacturing was going better than she'd expected. From the initial and wildly ambitious estimate that a vaccine candidate could be ready in 90 days, each new update seemed to shave off more time. The manufacturing team had canceled weekends and organized into shifts to make sure production kept moving ahead 24 hours a day. As February progressed, the expected late-April delivery date became early April, then late March, then mid-March. Suddenly Hamilton had weeks less time to get a clinical trial organized, find physicians and investigators to dose the product and recruit subjects to take it, write the protocol that dictated what the study would look like, and file paperwork with the FDA.

Once she did all that and the product materialized, the vaccine candidate would be ready to put into the arms of the first human test subjects. Traditionally, such trials proceeded in sequential phases: In the preclinical phase, the product would be tested in animals. A Phase I trial, with a small number of healthy human participants, would follow to test the product's safety in people. Phase II was for hunting in the subjects' blood for antibodies that would fight the virus, and to demonstrate that the vaccine had generated an immune response. In Phase III, the biggest trial, involving thousands of participants, researchers looked to see whether that immune response could actually prevent disease in the real world.

By February, Hamilton had gotten executive approval to take the project to Phase I and had enlisted government partners at the National Institutes of Health (NIH) to run the actual trial. But now that Phase I was bearing down, she had to think about what was supposed to happen afterward. Was she just trying to show what Moderna could do with its technology or was she actually trying to get a real vaccine, bring the company's first-ever product into large-scale trials and then to market? The virus had already been declared a public-health emergency in late January, but still no one knew if this was just a seasonal thing. The Zika experience of a false-start trial for a disappearing epidemic loomed in the background. Moderna's fundraising pitch to investors in February had been based almost entirely on the potential for its cytomegalovirus vaccine, ambitiously slated to enter Phase III trials sometime in 2020, and some investors had worried that the company risked getting distracted by its coronavirus research. The $500 million that came out of that endeavor wasn't intended to be a luxurious cushion for a shiny new product, but a necessary cash infusion for existing lines of research, some of them years in the making, for a company losing about $100 million per quarter.

For Hamilton, though, there was neither choice nor doubt: The team had to keep pushing ahead on coronavirus, even if it meant putting the entire company on the line. If this was going to be a pandemic, morally, they couldn't afford not to.

But for the company's board of directors—the uberbosses who told the executives what to do—this wasn't obvious. If Hamilton was going to get beyond Phase I, it wasn't enough to bring the gung-ho CEO and the hesitant president aboard. The board, specifically the part of it charged with overseeing the development pipeline start to finish, would determine whether Moderna's Covid vaccine lived or died.

She arrived at the board conference room on February 11 nervous but prepared, in her mild-mannered way, to do battle. The meeting space was on the floor of the building where many of the company's hot shots sat—the fancy part of the building, where visitors came, where everything was clean and crisp and white, where the offices and even the cubicles were encased in glass.

She had prepared a short slide deck, maybe too short, considering what was at stake: It was only about three slides long. She always worried, during presentations, that she was boring the audience, and anyway these were smart people who didn't need the basics explained to them. So the first slide showed where the virus was in the world at that point, which was still mostly in China—known U.S. cases had barely reached the double digits. The second listed the different ways the vaccine program could go over the next year, and the risks associated with each. The third showed the current status of the project, and what it would take to get a vaccine by the end of 2020 or early 2021. The whole presentation would last just 30 minutes.

Most of the eight people in front of her she'd never met

before. But she knew their reputations and the daunting concentration of achievements—academic decorations, pharmaceutical innovations, the launching of companies—and they also brought an alphabet's worth of degrees and prestigious affiliations: PhD, MD, FACP, FASCO. One person in particular, Moroccan-born American immunologist Moncef Slaoui, was a kind of professional model for Hamilton, though she didn't know him personally. He had led vaccine programs at the pharmaceutical giant GlaxoSmithKline, developing medicines for potential public-health threats, which was exactly what Hamilton thought Moderna should be doing.

And here she was with her master's degree and her slide deck, facing down their doubts.

Hamilton launched into her talk. To her mind, moving ahead would benefit the company no matter what happened. If the epidemic receded there would be no need to continue beyond Phase I, but then Moderna would at least have the beginnings of a vaccine to pull off the shelf in case the disease came back. Or they could even get from BARDA the government funding they needed to keep going, in a manner similar to their Zika program, if the government saw a potential resurgence as enough of a risk to invest against. Or the number of cases could explode, and Moderna could take trials all the way through Phase III, speed to an authorized vaccine, and debut its technology on the market by helping to stop a pandemic.

All this assumed the product actually worked. The alternative was to fail spectacularly as the world watched and hundreds of thousands of people died in America. There were plenty of examples of drugs that had looked promising in Phase II, only to show themselves ineffective in Phase III.

She noticed Moncef considering it all. "This makes sense," he said finally. "Let me just raise a few risks to you."

He knew from experience what happened when government money got involved: requirements, questions, and interested parties all multiplied. The company would be accountable not just to shareholders but to taxpayers, reporting to federal agencies hundreds of times bigger than the company itself, and fielding inquiries from politicians. The team could find itself rapidly overwhelmed just with keeping all the necessary actors informed and satisfied—and who were those, anyway? HHS? The CDC? The FDA? Were they even talking to the right people? Hamilton herself already knew what it was like to spend long nights racing to finish a BARDA proposal, only to wait weeks for it to be reviewed and returned with a battery of questions that, once answered, needed another few weeks' worth of review. Moncef's warnings suggested it could get much worse.

There was also the risk of an outright takeover of the company. In the event of a real pandemic, the government might use the Defense Production Act to force Moderna to halt all of its other work, abandon developing drugs for unmet needs around the world, and focus solely on the Covid vaccine. It was clear to Hamilton that Moncef wasn't sure it was worth it for the company. But Juan Andres, the technical operations chief in charge of getting supplies of the vaccine into trials, defended her. "We can do this," he said. "I've got a plan."

They continued to probe risks and concerns. When she'd answered all the questions she could, Hamilton left the room for the board members to continue their discussion without her. She

didn't wait for a formal green light. She just assumed she had it and
kept going.

■   ■   ■

The shutdown that came to Massachusetts in March was much less
a disruption for Hamilton than for most of her friends. She hadn't
socialized or gone to any bars or restaurants for weeks, consumed
as she was with getting the vaccine ready and moved into trials,
and now everyone she knew had to acclimate to a similar lonely
lifestyle. With everything closed, Hamilton had yet more time to
work, and so she did. She didn't fear missing out on St. Patrick's
Day or Cinco de Mayo or friends' barbecues, because those activities weren't options for anybody anymore. As painful as that reality
was for everyone, it required little further sacrifice from her. She
was stuck at a computer regardless.

    In practice her workdays resembled those of millions of home-
bound white-collar workers: She'd wake up and shuffle to her desk,
where she'd mostly stay until it was time to go to sleep again, eating
most of her meals there as she ran a gauntlet of emails and phone
calls and virtual meetings. In her case, though, all of these standard
office-drone exertions were directed toward one goal: To stop what
the World Health Organization was now calling a pandemic. It
wouldn't be enough for the manufacturing team just to produce
doses for clinical trials: If the vaccine worked, Moderna needed to
be ready to ship doses all over the country the second regulators
gave the okay. Hamilton's team was now chasing down suppliers
for raw materials and trying to secure the manufacturing capacity
to make vaccines on a scale Moderna had never before attempted.

In those early days in March she allowed herself a few indulgences. When she had time on the weekends, she'd join a video call with her husband and two other couples—far-flung friends, Johnny and Kadi in Virginia and Jess and Chase in the Netherlands, whom she and her husband knew from grad school and who were at this point really more like family. The six of them had traveled all over together, back when people traveled, and now settled for screen time and online tarot card readings—which, again, Hamilton knew were nonsense, if sometimes eerily prescient. Once, ahead of an important vaccine deadline, a card had signified that big things were coming. She played it cool for the sake of confidentiality. "Oh," she said. "Yep, mmhmm. Yes, they are."

Also, she'd never been much of a midweek drinker, but now that she was home all the time, she had to think of a way to break up the 12 hours of meetings. Kentucky-bred woman that she was, she opted for bourbon as she cleaned out her inbox.

Otherwise, she was pushing forward, navigating all the technical, bureaucratic, and financial hurdles involved in attempting a feat that neither her company nor any other, anywhere, had tried before. Regulators hadn't even had time to come up with guidance for pursuing a Covid vaccine; Hamilton and her team were flying blind, trying to design manufacturing practices and clinical trials to conform to rules that didn't even exist yet. There was always the chance that the FDA could swoop in months down the road and snarl up the whole process with dozens of new requirements.

But Hamilton couldn't worry about that now. In April, she secured a promise for close to $500 million in BARDA funding. In May, Moderna announced hopeful interim results from Phase I trials: The first eight human volunteers had exhibited immune responses to the shots, two apiece spaced four weeks apart, and their bodies had started pumping out antibodies that could defend against a real infection. Meanwhile, for mice injected with the vaccine and then deliberately infected with SARS-CoV-2, Moderna's shot had stopped the virus colonizing their lungs.

On the strength of that data, the company raised a further billion-plus dollars in May from investors anxious for a Covid silver bullet and grasping at the good news.

At that point, it was clear that Moderna, and specifically Hamilton, were entirely on the hook to see this thing through. There would be no stopping after Phase I. And the government support was great to have, but still forthcoming—it was meant as a reimbursement, which meant Moderna had to blow out its own bank account before seeing a dime's worth of that help, which even then could take months to show up.

Because if in fact the vaccine worked, the company would eventually need to crank out something like a billion doses; which meant they'd have to start now, before even knowing whether the vaccine was effective; which meant they might just be wasting a billion dollars of their own money on a massive stockpile of drugs that didn't even work; and, oh, by the way, the disease could still disappear in the summer. So maybe, at Hamilton's insistence, they were all on the verge of bankrupting the company and destroying everything they'd built and all the programs they'd been working on for years.

But maybe the country and the world needed them to take that chance. So Moderna blew through its cash. The government could show up when it caught up.

■ ■ ■

Around the same time, on May 15, the Trump administration announced a new program to coordinate among all the federal agencies that had a hand in vaccine development or oversight, fund and speed the production of the vaccine, and help soften the massive financial risks that vaccine-seeking companies such as Moderna were taking on. Its name, Operation Warp Speed, bespoke its ambitions—even though Hamilton and her team had already spent four months chasing a vaccine by the time OWS even formed.

The administration was willing to put an enormous amount of money and muscle behind vaccine research, especially compared with its laissez-faire approach to promoting shorter-term mitigation measures. But the vaccine seemed to hold out the promise of fixing everything all at once: It demanded no consistent behaviors such as hand-washing and mask-wearing and keeping distance from others, no tiresome habits for everyone to do, every day. Just a little stick or two in the arm could give back American life as it once was. You could go to a restaurant or even a bar. You could shake a stranger's hand or hug your grandchildren.

That was the hope, anyway, for the administration, for millions of Americans, and certainly for Hamilton. But alongside that hope walked fear. It wasn't just the newness and stunning speed of the proposed mRNA approach—if it worked.

First, there was the question, prompted by suspected repeat Covid infections reported out of China and Japan as early as February, of whether a practice infection via a vaccine could really prevent a real infection. Isolated accounts of people enduring the illness more than once suggested anecdotally that this wasn't necessarily a disease like chicken pox, which a person might contract a single time and then be immune from forevermore. This new coronavirus could behave more like coronaviruses that cause the common cold, which were capable of recurring more than once in the same people, whose immune defenses challenged the virus for a time and then stood down and left the body vulnerable to the virus's return.

If that was the case, and if actual infection didn't leave behind enough or strong enough antibodies to prevent a recurrence of infection, then what did that mean for a vaccine? Or did those who re-contracted Covid just not have enough exposure the first time to develop a robust immune response? Hamilton feared the possibilities, but there was really no answer except to test and measure over time the consistency of antibody response to a vaccine candidate.

The scientific problems were difficult enough, but there were also the questions of politics and psychology. Suppose the FDA felt political pressure to approve a vaccine below typical standards of safety and efficacy—not at all an idle possibility in a presidential election year with a bitterly divided population sick of pandemic living. Federal agencies did not have an exquisite pandemic track record to begin with, starting with the CDC's testing fumble, when the agency distributed faulty tests around the country in early February and then took weeks to fix the problem. On March 20, the president had promoted the anti-malarial drug hydroxychloroquine to battle the coronavirus. In late March, the FDA authorized the drug for emergency use for COVID-19 patients, citing a reasonable belief that it could be effective on the basis of anecdotal data and noting there really wasn't time to conduct proper trials in the pandemic. In June, the

FDA rescinded the authorization, stating that it was unlikely to be an effective treatment for Covid and that, moreover, "in light of ongoing serious cardiac adverse events and other potential serious side effects," the risks outweighed the benefits of using the drug. It had taken nearly three months for the agency to reverse its position.

Additional screw-ups certainly weren't out of the question. Suppose large numbers of people were immunized with a vaccine that wasn't effective, and then went about their lives as before, assuming they couldn't spread the disease. And then what if all those crowded house parties celebrating the end of the pandemic actually ended up giving it a new life?

And would this whole "Warp Speed" branding, borrowed from *Star Trek* and presumably intended to foster hope that the nation could get out of this soon, instead seed the impression that the whole process was rushed and the product unsafe? It was one thing to be sick in a hospital and sign up for an emergency experimental treatment, tolerating a certain amount of risk for a shot at getting better. But vaccines were meant to be taken by millions of healthy people. Trump himself had, prior to becoming president, raised questions about vaccine safety in general, and alleged a link between vaccines and autism. In the spring of 2019, the United States experienced a measles outbreak in several states, and the president seemed to reverse himself, urging people to get their shots and declaring that vaccinations were important.

Roughly a year later, he had set the federal government and a herd of private companies on an all-out gallop for a new vaccine that so many hoped could halt the pandemic—and many others didn't trust.

The Paramedic

March 28–April 19, 2020

No matter how soon the vaccine came, though, it would be too late to stop the carnage in New York, where Paul and his crew of Coloradans were getting ready to throw themselves into the crucible. First, though, they had some down time after they arrived on March 28, and they spent the evening playing tourists in a shut-down city, on a then still-rare Saturday night when, anywhere you looked in Manhattan, there was nothing much to do. What they could do, the whole dozen of them, was wedge themselves into their ambulances and cruise around to observe from their windows the strange stillness of the avenues, the streets cleared of their crowds, the garish screens and posters of Times Square hawking denim and cell-phone plans to no one. Naturally, they had to avoid the subway system, and they also had to pay attention to where they parked. (New York City cops, they were advised, didn't care that they were hero helpers from out of town—they'd still hand out tickets.)

Paul sat in the back of one of the ambulances with four others, enduring the young-people music pumping loud from the front. The radio blasted out "Empire State of Mind," Jay-Z and Alicia Keys's love letter to a thrilling city that looked nothing like the ghost town Paul and his new friends now drove through. *There's nothing you can't do, now you're in New York.* Paul was much more into bagpipes than rap but was having a surreal kind of fun. Dinner was takeout from Katz's Delicatessen on the Lower East Side of Manhattan, famed for its towering pastrami-on-rye sandwiches at the astonishing price of about $25.

The crew made another stop near the 9/11 memorial and got out of their trucks to walk around. Just a year before a new monument to first responders had opened near the site, six granite slabs honoring the 343 firefighters Paul often kept in mind who perished the day of the attacks. September 11, 2001, was the deadliest day U.S. firefighters had ever seen, with many crushed after charging into the towers to rescue those trapped inside, right before the towers collapsed entirely. Hundreds more had died in the years that followed from exposure to the site's toxins, which burrowed into their lungs and attacked them slowly from the inside.

Much of the memorial was blocked off, so they couldn't get close enough to read the inscription:

> *Here we honor the tens of thousands*
> *From across America and around the world*
> *Who came to help and to heal*
> *Whose selflessness and resolve*

Perseverance and courage
Renewed the spirit of a grieving city
Gave hope to the nation
And inspired the world.

■   ■   ■

In the absence of New York's normal throng of sightseers and convention-goers, the city's hotels sat largely empty, staff members furloughed or laid off. At the same time, though, out-of-town volunteers such as Paul were descending on the city, local medical workers were trying to avoid going home for fear of exposing their families, and the infected but not hospitalized also needed space away from family. So New York's hotels began apportioning their empty rooms to people like this, which is how Paul ended up at a Sheraton in Queens.

It was normally an airport hotel, wedged into a busy block in Flushing about a 10-minute drive from LaGuardia; you could look up from the sidewalk outside the Sheraton and see the white fish-bellies of descending planes. The FDNY's EMS Battalion 52 station sat a block over. The neighborhood, sometimes called the "Chinese Manhattan" for its predominant ethnic group and relentless bustle, was usually packed with people, and the dim sum and dumpling joints did a brisk business. Covid, though, had spooked the residents, who were early to take the disease seriously as horrifying news flowed in from relatives or friends in China. By mid-March, masks had begun to appear on the faces bobbing along the streets, though the CDC wouldn't recommend their use among the general public until April. Some 20 Chinese grocery stores had shut down voluntarily, despite having the option to stay open as essential businesses. Business owners in Flushing had been early to install Plexiglass barriers and hand out masks, but now people were simply too afraid to go to work.

When Paul checked in, the guest list at the Sheraton, a frequent commuter crash pad offering space for conferences and weddings, was basically all emergency workers. More than 100 were there from all over the country, many of them bunking with roommates, like a college dorm where the campus was catastrophe.

So far New York State had suffered more than 1,200 deaths relating to the virus, and local officials were darkly warning that the worst was yet to come. As the president voiced his hope that the country would vanquish the virus by Easter, hundreds of people were being admitted to New York City hospitals with Covid-like symptoms every day.

In parallel, some 250 ambulances and 500 first responders were streaming into the city to help, hauling their vehicles from Tennessee, Virginia, California, Pennsylvania, and elsewhere at the behest of the Federal Emergency Management Agency. They filtered through the check-in at the FDNY's training academy in Fort Totten, Queens, where on March 31 New York's fire commissioner Daniel Nigro delivered a pep talk, declaring he almost couldn't believe so many people would show up for New Yorkers' dark hour. But he was looking around and saw that it was a real thing. "Thank each and every one of you for coming from where you are to help us," he said. "When the time comes that your communities need help, I hope we're in a position here where we can reciprocate, and help you the same way."

About 85 refrigerated trucks were also on the way, for the people no one could save.

There wasn't much time for Paul to spend hanging out in the Sheraton. After his own Fort Totten check-in, he was assigned to a five-ambulance team—Strike Team 19—which was set to take the 9:00 a.m. to 9:00 p.m. shift. This meant a 3:30 a.m. wakeup time to eat a hotel breakfast and get ready for a shuttle, which took Paul and other emergency workers to their ambulances at 5:30 a.m. to check them over and make sure they had all the supplies they needed. A variety of needles, two or three sizes for each type. Barely pronounceable tools such as the sphygmomanometer, better known as a blood-pressure cuff. Bandages, defibrillators, oxygen devices, restraints, obstetrical equipment—everything required to stop bleeding, start a heartbeat, deliver a baby, or perform any number of minor miracles without the resources of a hospital.

Queens was still dark on the first morning Paul's shuttle carried him over the Whitestone Bridge spanning the East River, past the golf course near the water with its "TRUMP LINKS" sign visible from the highway, and to the Bronx Zoo. The parking lot on the southwest corner of the park was being overtaken by ambulances ready to shoot out across the city's five boroughs. In normal times the blacktop was accustomed to throngs of sensible sedans and minivans on pleasant-day family outings, as the grass slowly reasserted itself through thickening cracks in the asphalt. Now it was turning into a small city of hundreds of purring white or blue trucks, interspersed with tents and porta-potties and snack trucks, and games people brought as if on a camping trip: badminton sets and Frisbees and footballs to toss around.

The zoo was also where, incidentally, a four-year-old tiger named Nadia would test positive for the coronavirus, adding a cat victim to the many thousands of people sick or dying in the Bronx.

But at least in that parking lot, it seemed like the whole country had come to help. Culture shock notwithstanding: Some were perplexed by the bacon-egg-and-cheese-on-a-roll bodega sandwich, some hadn't planned for the chill and had failed to bring jackets, some even had trouble with the vocabulary (an ambulance, in New York EMS parlance, was a "bus," not a "rig").

Paul's first 12-hour shift wound up lasting 42 hours, which he mainly spent waiting for things to happen while administrators figured out how exactly to manage this colossal deployment. He and Alissa bitched amicably about being made to stand around, but FEMA was trying to put together an essentially brand-new ambulance service of hundreds in the space of a few days. The ambulance crews hung out with each other or napped in their trucks. In the chaos of stitching together a wide variety of emergency services, coming from vastly different local contexts, no one noticed for nearly two days that Strike Team 19 hadn't been relieved. But then, finally, the shift ended, and they went back to the hotel.

Which was around the time the calls started flooding in for the out-of-towners. Paul barely had time to get back to his room and take off his boots before the instruction came to get back downstairs and back on the shuttle; he was needed again at the Bronx Zoo, where he and the team spent the next 30 hours.

This time they didn't wait around. The job was basically infinite—call after call to hospital after hospital, where Paul and the others would retrieve stricken patients from overwhelmed wards and ferry them to places with more space. "Hospital decompression," it was called, as if you were twisting the cap off a shaken-up Coca-Cola bottle to let out the fizz. Even the places with more space threatened to run out of it; Governor Cuomo declared the state could ultimately need 140,000 hospital beds—with only 53,000 available. The Javits Center on Manhattan's West Side, a glittery glass behemoth on the Hudson that should have been hosting the New York International Auto Show that time of year, had been shut down and repurposed as a mammoth field hospital. In a matter of weeks, the Army Corps of Engineers and its contractors outfitted the nearly 2-million-square-foot expo center with 2,500 beds, and planned to set up similar makeshift medical facilities in unused dorms, hotels, and convention centers around the country. State leaders throughout the nation were watching projections of the virus's spread and fearing their own hospitals could soon be as overwhelmed as New York's. The Navy sent a hospital ship, the USNS *Comfort*, to Pier 90 to float on the Hudson River about a mile north.

The original plan had been for both the transformed Javits Center and the *Comfort* to take only non-Covid patients, to allow hospitals to focus on pandemic cases without abandoning everyone else needing medical care. But Covid soon overtook those plans. Hospitals' overwhelming need was for Covid bedspace, and Javits and the *Comfort*, in refusing Covid patients, were initially barely taking in anyone. (Many injuries, it turned out, could be avoided if you never left home.) So both wound up as Covid treatment centers, too.

Elsewhere, extreme chaos stalked every corridor and trauma bay Paul visited. Maybe 15 or 20 people on ventilators in any given emergency room, people lying on their backs, on their stomachs, fighting for breath. Multiple ventilator alarms going off at once, a ghoulish music box, signifying something wrong with the breathing aids, too much air pressure, not enough, a leak or a blockage or a spasming patient. Some ventilators were being shared among multiple patients.

Nurses were overwhelmed and exhausted and no one seemed to know where, exactly, the patients were that the decompression ambulances were supposed to take away. Paul had to walk sideways through a thicket of beds, reading footboard tape to try to find whichever patient he'd been sent for; move other beds blocking the path to the exit; and finally wheel the patient back out to the ambulance. Sometimes just finding the patient could take an hour. At Elmhurst a patient awaiting transfer died before an ambulance could get there; at Flushing Medical Center an EMT couldn't get a cot all the way through the hospital door, because even the hallway was full.

The worst part was knowing that, even when a patient did manage to get transferred somewhere with a little more space, maybe making one small dent in a hospital's overcrowding, there would soon be another to take that person's place. There were patients who died waiting for transfers, and patients who were clearly not going to make it after transfer but needed to be moved to make room for others with a better shot at survival.

Back at the Bronx Zoo, getting dinner from the food trucks or waiting for the next call, Paul got to know his new band of brothers and sisters. Strike Team 19's leader, Jerrod Estes, had arrived from central Illinois, where he owned his own ambulance company, and had brought some of his employees to New York. He was himself a family man and a former firefighter, decades Paul's junior, and as they got to swapping stories, Paul seemed to have an inexhaustible supply of adventures to describe. A colleague back in Aurora had once joked that Paul was a "shit-magnet" who seemed to respond to all the abnormal 911 calls, the summer-night gunshot victims, the septic patients in their eighties brought in from a nursing home, people on the verge of death he'd just drop off in the ER. His had been one of the first ambulances on the scene when a gunman killed a dozen people in an Aurora movie theater in 2012.

Paul's stories became so infamous that some of the younger members of his Bronx team would jokingly groan or pretend to hold their ears when he launched into one of them. His firehouse mustache was also a frequent object of gentle ribbing: "Hey, Paul, it's not the 1980s anymore." The days were frequently cold, in that way New York Aprils have of shambling noncommittally toward spring, and Paul wore a beanie hat that was slightly too small and kept creeping up above his ears. He spoke with pride about his kids and grandkids, and Jerrod sought his counsel on the family strains of the job, and the struggle to be there for one's own loved ones while trying to also be there for strangers in crisis. They mused about what they would do when it was all over, and Paul invited Jerrod to come to Colorado someday, where he could show him around the firehouses and they'd have a barbecue.

It was hard to imagine when this all would be over.

The days trudged by. Paul's team got switched to the night shift, 7:00 p.m. to 7:00 a.m., which effectively meant 5:30 p.m. to 9:00 a.m., with commuting and ambulance prep time. He was getting used to it, this relentless pace that he'd sought for himself all along. The need for him was so obviously great, and for all the lives lost, he knew he was saving some who wouldn't otherwise have made it. That was worth it. It was worth it to make the overwhelmed hospital workers' jobs just the tiniest increment easier, and certainly worth it to help relieve the pressure on his brethren New York paramedics and EMTs.

In the Aurora medical system, everybody knew Paul's name, by virtue of the decades he'd spent in the community. But the camaraderie of a deployment like this developed rapidly and reached deeply. He now saw many faces he recognized among the paramedics and EMTs at various hospitals around the city and at the Javits Center where he stopped frequently with patients. He joined a text chain with the others from Colorado, including Alissa and another guy from Colorado Springs, Royce Davis, and they traded stories and checked in with one another in the Bronx Zoo parking lot.

Out on his rounds, bemasked and swaddled in protective gear, Paul had been forced to obscure his most recognizable feature, his voluptuous 1980s 'stache. Yet he retained a smirk that reached his eyes over his mask. And that, as they passed one another in hospital hallways or through the Javits Center's maze of beds, was a source of reassurance to some of his colleagues. *Don't worry*, he seemed to say. *If you see me worry, then you can go ahead and worry.*

■   ■   ■

Then he started to feel poorly.

Alissa was on Strike Team 18, parked next to Paul's unit and working the same shifts, spending time with him on the lot during downtime. She'd noticed near the middle of April that he was looking tired, and it made sense: This was tiring work. It seemed to be getting to Paul a bit faster than the others, but then again, Paul was both older and more fanatical about work than most of his peers—all of whom were fanatical enough to have driven from their own homes to ride their ambulances around a strange city gripped by sickness.

Health checks every 12 hours were mandatory for the emergency workers. Getting off the shuttle bus from the hotel to the Bronx Zoo, Paul would join the line to the medical trailer for a temperature and symptom check. An app collected everyone's FEMA unit number, name, phone number, and temperature reading, then offered a checklist of symptoms to enter if applicable: cough, difficulty breathing, loss of sense of taste and smell. That way, someone with the onsite medical team could come and find anyone on the lot if something was wrong, as an infection could spread rapidly and easily among the emergency workers—who shared hotels and shuttle buses, drove their ambulances in pairs, and lounged together in the parking lot between calls. Otherwise, there was an option at the bottom of the list to report feeling great.

"Feeling great" in that environment wasn't really an option, no matter how physically healthy one was. The first responders were seeing things they'd never seen before, some of them in long careers and some of them in short ones. One former Marine who'd spent years on overseas deployments declared the experience worse than his time in the military; one twenty-something from California with no prior experience answering 911 calls was found by a colleague balled up on a subway platform, crying, because he'd just worked his first cardiac arrest.

Even if someone felt a slight cough or tickle in the throat coming on, it was easy enough to chalk that up to fatigue. A few people had already wound up in quarantine, but no one wanted to be the guy who potentially lost days of work, forced to rest, because of symptoms that might turn out to be nothing. Still less did any of the EMTs and paramedics want to take up hospital space in an overwhelmed system when they were specifically there trying to make things easier for local health workers.

Alissa was dealing with kidney pains one shift when she ran into Paul at the medical trailer. She asked him how he was doing. "If I could get some sleep, I might feel better," he responded.

"Yeah, well, we all want to sleep," she said. "Do you mean you're not sleeping at all?"

He told her he pretty much had to sit up straight to sleep, and that he just hadn't felt good for a few days. Alissa was sorry to hear it. She figured he was just being a typical medical guy, the type of person who would just keep showing up to do the job. The two of them had discussed their plans for after their two-week deployment ended, and whether they'd take the option to stay for another stint in the city. No matter how tired Paul was, Alissa could tell he wasn't going home.

"I'm staying," he'd said.

Now the two of them were well into their third week in New York as other colleagues prepared to head home. She still had no reason to doubt he'd keep staying until the job was done. She left him there in the medical trailer, expecting to see him soon.

The Nurse

Testing Shortage

March 29–April 20, 2020

ELSEWHERE IN THE BRONX, Michelle was watching her parents with a persistent, fearful refrain running through her mind: *Please just let it be a cold.* Papo had the worst of it, whatever it was. He'd worked for the Metropolitan Transportation Authority for more than 30 years, and he now manned a booth at the Bedford Park Boulevard subway stop, where the No. 4 train came and went. New York's transit workers were getting hit hard by the coronavirus, with thousands sickened and dozens killed by early April. And Papo was staying home now, with a fever that just wouldn't quit.

He was squarely in the "high-risk" category—he suffered from hemolytic anemia, an autoimmune disorder in which the immune system destroys red blood cells so fast that the bone marrow can't keep up a proper supply. In other words, he was "immunocompromised," precisely the kind of person who needed to take extra pains to avoid the virus and, as an essential worker, precisely the kind who couldn't. Michelle had already spent several days in the ICU watching what the disease could do even to healthier bodies. And what if she herself had brought the disease home? And what if he ended up in the hospital, where she knew there was a high likelihood that the caregivers themselves might be hurting their patients?

She blamed herself. If this was Covid, if she had it too, she thought she must have gotten it from reusing her mask so many times, storing it in a paper bag and then digging it out to use again, with who knew what infectious pathogens lurking in there and clinging to the mask. But maybe there was still a chance this wasn't Covid.

By then, at least, the family had decided that no matter what precautions they took, it was too dangerous for Grandma to stay with them. And Grandma, despite her dementia, knew well enough what was happening as Covid crashed into Montefiore and the surrounding neighborhood. She'd watched the coverage on *Univision Canal 6* and saw that the world was changing but not yet how it would upend her own life. Though to Michelle's eyes, the station's newscasters, like many other people, seemed to be playing down the real risks.

For a time, Michelle had tried not to get anywhere near Grandma, which was difficult and sad. Grandma had fallen a few times in the preceding months, and Carmen at times would grow strict and impatient with her to sit still, eat her food, drink her water. Sometimes in those moments, Grandma would, like a child in trouble, mournfully reach for Michelle as a source of safety from her daughter's anger. And Michelle would just as mournfully deny that to her—*No puedo tocarte.* I can't touch you.

Grandma knew the rituals, even if she sometimes forgot the

restrictions, and Michelle and her other family members told her directly and repeatedly that if someone in the house got sick, Grandma was going to have to leave. No one wanted to wrench an old woman with dementia from her home, but no one wanted to kill her, either.

No puede quedarte acqui. Tu te puede morir.

A few days before Michelle's worst shift on March 28, the family moved Grandma down the street to an uncle's apartment.

Now, just home from that shift and suffering from her own symptoms, Michelle was putting an oximeter onto her dad's fingertip to read the health of his blood. His oxygen level was at 87 percent. Panic swept over her. She feared she'd fled Covid at the hospital only to find it at home. She called out sick the next day. She didn't know what was wrong with her, but she had to find out for sure what was wrong with her parents. They needed tests.

The nation's crisis was tightening its grip on Michelle's individual life.

Montefiore had set up a testing center in a big white tent outside its emergency room, in an effort to limit traffic into the hospital. It had been two and a half months since the virus had arrived in the United States, and more than two weeks since the president had declared its spread to be a national emergency. And still the country lacked enough tests even to identify all the disease's victims. In February, during the weeks when state and local labs were relying on faulty tests from the CDC, regulators were also hamstringing their ability to develop alternatives. To conserve scarce tests, the CDC had also early on restricted who could be tested, emphasizing travel history. In January, testing was limited to only those who had traveled to Wuhan; in early February, to those with severe respiratory illness who had been to China; at the end of February, to those who had been to other hot-spot countries or were hospitalized with respiratory illness; and finally, on March 5, the CDC loosened the guidelines to allow physicians to administer tests at their discretion. Around the same time, Cuomo had announced what for the United States was an ambitious goal, to conduct 1,000 tests a day statewide. South Korea, with a population two and half times the size that of New York State, was by then doing 10 times the number of daily tests.

Consequently Montefiore, too, was rationing tests just as it was rationing protective equipment. But it seemed reasonable to Michelle that the hospital would test one of its own, knowing how much time she'd spent near Covid patients—and as for her parents, well, it might be because of Montefiore that they were in this predicament in the first place. Surely that counted for something.

Michelle staggered out of the apartment and into the family car, pulling it around to the entrance of her apartment building where she watched her parents guide each other carefully across the sidewalk, looking to her more like a couple in their eighties than their sixties. She drove them the short distance to the hospital and left them in the dark cold of the hospital's underground ambulance parking by the testing tent while she ran, as best she could manage with her labored breath, to her manager on the second floor to plead for help. "My parents are downstairs," she wheezed. "I'm sick. I need them tested. Governor Cuomo said that if you need a test, people are being tested. Is there any muscle you can use to try to get them tested?" Her boss told her to go back downstairs and explain to the critical-care manager there that she was a medical ICU nurse.

When Michelle rejoined her parents, nurses were already assessing them, taking their blood pressure and asking questions, but one of them informed Michelle that the hospital didn't have any tests to spare. Most likely her parents had Covid, Michelle's colleague told her, but they should just go home and quarantine.

Michelle was embarrassed, not just to beg but to ask for something on the basis of her position that other people couldn't get. It flew in the face of her values to ask for VIP care. But this was her own hospital, where she'd brought her own family, and she didn't know what else to do; her dad was not well. "My dad has an auto-immune disorder. He has hypertension," she said. The governor had just been bragging about New York state's aggressive testing at a news conference. "What's wrong? Why isn't this happening?" Her family was suffering, and now the hospital was telling them they weren't even entitled to know the cause. Michelle loved the ER nurses, she didn't blame them for what was happening, she knew that they were working under impossible conditions. It was just that it shouldn't be impossible for Michelle to take care of her own family.

Maybe 10 other people were there waiting for tests; some coughing, sitting as far away from each other as they could; some with masks and some without. A young woman paced back and forth shouting her irritation into a cell phone about how long she'd been waiting there, every once in a while pulling off her mask as if to shout better.

The mask thing made Michelle nervous, but she couldn't bring herself to get angry. *How can I be mad at you? I'm mad at the same thing. I'm about to pull off* my *fucking mask.* If her parents didn't already have Covid, they could get it today, sitting here in the chill of what was effectively a parking garage basement with so many sick others.

The best Michelle's colleague could offer was a chest X-ray for her dad, to see if his lungs were showing signs of pneumonia—but given the hospital's crush of patients, it would take three or four hours to get the procedure. Michelle knew the hospital well enough to know that the nurse was telling the truth.

She was fatigued from disease, from worry, from effort, from defeat. She turned around and saw her mother standing not far behind her, short of breath, getting ready to argue. She saw Carmen's fingers going up, preparing to point and wag like she was about to demand to talk to corporate or whatever. She saw her dad sitting in the back of a tent, slumped over. She made a decision.

I gotta get the fuck out of here.

"Mami please. Please please please. You don't have it in you to fight this right now, and we're not *going* to fight this right now, because I'm not fighting against the same people that I protect. We gotta go." She was getting upset, and she did not want to get upset with people who were just trying to do their jobs.

So she grabbed her folks and went home and said a prayer, an Our Father surrounded by a few apologies for not tapping in sooner. "It's your girl Michelle. I know we haven't spoke in a while . . ." She was a Catholic out of practice, and she thought it probably best to lay some groundwork in case God didn't remember who she was. Then she got to begging that her parents wouldn't die.

■   ■   ■

It was the worst at night. Michelle was scared to go to sleep because she knew people with Covid would sometimes go to sleep and never wake up. But she always did wake up, feeling flashes of heat and covered in sweat, her chest tight, whether from the illness or from anxiety she couldn't really tell. Michelle's mom knew someone at a nearby urgent-care clinic, which was doing five tests a day, so the day after failing to get tests at Montefiore her parents managed to snag some and confirm what they already knew.

Michelle was nervous about her parents getting worse and being the only person there to take care of them, so she set an alarm on her phone to make sure to check on them every two or three hours during the night. She would listen to her father snoring and in each scraping, rattling breath she heard a warning that her parents might not make it. Her dad had sleep apnea, hence the snoring, which was really the sound of his brain potentially being deprived of oxygen.

During the day she made sure they drank a lot of tea and took steam baths, leaning their heads over pots of steaming water draped in towels to keep the mist inside. She had no appetite herself for anything but tea and soup. Just walking around the house left her exhausted.

Yet she knew that a few blocks away, her hospital was getting inundated with patients, her colleagues were being worked past their limits, and she wasn't there to help. Staff members were dropping; the first week Michelle called out sick, she was one of maybe five or six people she knew of that did so, then another five left the following week. Some were getting hospitalized with critical symptoms. James Goodrich, a 73-year-old pediatric neurosurgeon at Montefiore, a Vietnam Marine veteran famous for his skill at separating conjoined twins with fused brains, died of complications from COVID-19 on March 30.

Her friends were in danger, her family was in danger, she herself was in danger, and she was powerless to help. She barely had the power to fill her own lungs. A manager called Michelle several days into her absence, in Michelle's mind to pressure her to come back to work—the manager had already returned after being sick the prior week. She felt guilty. And so very, very weak.

■   ■   ■

She dreaded going back to work. It had now been 14 days since Michelle first started showing symptoms, and she knew that Monte was short-staffed on a good day, and that the hospital hadn't seen a good day for weeks now. She was much better than she had been, but still wasn't herself. Her parents' fevers had dropped, though they, too, were still struggling. Her brain felt foggy and she wasn't sure she'd be able to exhibit the reflexes her job required. As a nurse you needed to be on your game, always ready to jump or run to the bedside of someone who needed intervention.

She knew also that there would be no room to make mistakes. In normal times, you could ask a coworker to keep an eye on your patients for an extra hour if you didn't feel well and needed to go lie down. Nurses looked out for each other that way. But now everyone was overworked and everyone needed to be there to hold things together.

So Michelle trudged up the hill to the hospital on April 12, carrying a towering stack of anxieties. She recognized this feeling of dread, though it was rare for her: She'd felt something like it when she'd first started in the medical ICU and wondered if she'd made the right decision, and another time when she'd walked into her first night shift and realized she'd never before stayed up from 7 o'clock at night to 7 o'clock in the morning. But this time was different, because she was now fearful about her own abilities. She'd be trying to pull as many patients as she could back from the Covid abyss she'd just spent weeks staring into, having barely recovered herself and still worrying about whether her parents would escape the disease's death grip. She prayed she wasn't still infectious.

She pushed past the dread. She knew the alternative was to stay paralyzed by it. *Fuck it*, she thought. *What else is going to happen to me at this point?*

For starters, her bosses were sending her to another makeshift ICU. And on her first day back, she was going to be in charge of the nurses there.

In her absence the hospital had opened a new ICU in an unused space in the building, one that nurses had long agitated to open for regular patients, given that the hospital had been cramming stretchers into hallways before Covid had even appeared in Wuhan. The nurses' conditions had improved slightly in the two weeks Michelle had been gone. More masks were available, so that now a nurse could use one mask per day versus one mask per week.

Other features of the crisis had not changed. The hospital didn't have enough critical-care doctors for all the critical patients, so the attending physicians in the unit came from other disciplines such as dermatology and gynecology, not typically associated with caring for ventilated patients. Michelle was the only ICU nurse in the ward—the others were medical–surgical, or med-surge, nurses, who generally took care of patients on their way into or out of surgery. Those patients were typically stable, getting ready to go home; maybe one or two of them had an intravenous drip for antibiotics. But ICU nurses liked to joke that they could get four or six IV medications into a patient and always know which medicine was going through which tube. Med-surge nurses only occasionally worked with patients on ventilators. They did not have Michelle's level of experience caring for patients on the verge of death, though they were accumulating more and more the longer the crisis went on.

Michelle's new unit had about a dozen patients and four nurses, including Michelle, which meant three patients apiece. Nearly all were on ventilators.

Ventilators were extremely sensitive machines, difficult to manage and prone to sounding alarms at any minor disturbance—by design, as even slight variations in their settings could severely injure or even kill a patient. Ordinarily it could take more than half an hour to get the settings on a ventilator just right for one patient, calibrating pressure and oxygen and breath speed, but each additional patient left less time for the others and less expertise with the machine to spare. If someone was waking up from sedation and coughed, it could set off an alarm. If a nurse was passing by or adjusting a patient's medications and bumped the machine, it could start wailing a protest.

Michelle had been through this many times, and she knew the important thing was not to panic. The important thing was to be

quiet, take a breath, and listen to whether there was air rushing
through a tube that had been disconnected or suction for mucus
buildup in the tubes, and then call for a respiratory therapist or a
physician if troubleshooting steps didn't quiet the alarm. She wasn't
sure how comfortable her new team was with any of this, so she
resolved to try to keep an eye on all 12 patients, checking on one
after the other, and then starting over again at the top. The problem was that she, too, was at a disadvantage, because this unit was
full of strange, government-issued ventilators with unfamiliar con-
trols and no screens to help identify problems.

And she wasn't prepared for what she saw among the patients.

She could tell at first glance that the patients' beds weren't
meant for prolonged stays on a ventilator. They were stretchers, not
real beds; she heard from another nurse they were there because
proper beds wouldn't fit through the door to the unit. As she
turned a patient for bathing, she saw the patient's bedsores that had
developed from prolonged pressure, where bones poked into the
skin. The sores were deep and raw and disgusting, another indignity inflicted on stricken patients fighting for their lives.

Michelle started to cry. *God help us.*

God help us all.

■   ■   ■

That was how the pandemic's cruelest month in New York City
began for Michelle. The state's death toll kept ticking up, surpassing that of 9/11 by April 3, and more than doubling it by the middle
of the month. The governor ordered that all of New York's flags fly
at half-mast, displaying the state's constant state of mourning. And

with the state then reporting more coronavirus cases than any *country* outside the United States, aerial photographs of Hart Island, a strip of land off the Bronx that had longed served as a graveyard for the city's poor and unclaimed dead, showed the fresh trenches of new mass graves.

At Montefiore's Moses campus, Michelle was preoccupied with her parents' health as she tried to get through work as best as she could. The hospital was absorbing more than triple its normal volume of critical patients, and Michelle ran through day after day on adrenaline-fueled autopilot.

Her friend Taeler, a former traveling nurse who had done a stint in New York in 2016, fallen in love with the city, and decided to stay, called her one night and cried for hours into a smartphone screen, drinking a bottle of champagne by herself. The two had been close for years and had shared a last, pre-shutdown bar visit together prior to St. Patrick's Day, at the Bronx Ale House where they'd listened to the Hudson Valley Regional Police Irish band play their bagpipes and drums. After that they'd stopped hanging out in person because they didn't want to infect each other. That night on the phone, Taeler confessed to her feelings of helplessness—as an ICU nurse she prided herself on helping people die if necessary, as that was part of life after all, but she had never let anybody die alone until Covid. She'd seen nurses who had served decades, whose strength she admired, break down from the relentlessness of the disease.

Michelle had seen many of the same things, and if she couldn't offer reassurance that it was going to get better, she at least had all her own versions of the same stories. Taeler had tried different meds on a patient as his blood pressure dropped, realized there was nothing to be done, and stood nearby as a doctor called the patient's wife on his cell phone because he was running out of time to find the iPad that now accompanied the dying at their bedsides instead of their actual loved ones. Taeler had listened as the dying man's wife screamed into the phone, and as his child, who couldn't have been more than four or five years old, cried. *Daddy? Daddy? Why aren't you home?* There were too many dead now to remember them all: Once a 12-bed unit had lost seven patients overnight, and she'd heard of coworkers coming back in the morning to find that all their patients from the previous shift were dead. But Taeler thought about this one man all the time.

Like Michelle, though, Taeler had also seen miracles. And this had always been a big part of what it meant to be an ICU nurse— either helping patients die peacefully or, in the best cases, aiding their escape from death. There was nothing like seeing someone almost die and then, somehow, get back up and walk. Michelle's former patient, the nurse she had coaxed off the ventilator, was back on the job caring for other patients. One of Taeler's patients had been on the verge of being transferred to palliative care for an eas- ier death when she'd suddenly woken up, and had been transferred to rehab instead.

At some point, hospital staff at Montefiore had decided to cele- brate these victories by playing "Empire State of Mind" over the PA system, so that everyone could hear it when people got extubated or discharged. For Taeler this was a sign of hope in the hospital, even when she couldn't see it herself. *There's nothing you can't do.*

Michelle took a darker view, because, like Taeler, every day she faced the many things she couldn't do. She also knew that, once freed from the ventilator, there was a decent chance a patient would have to go back on it, and what was the proper song for that?

Sometime in April, she heard about the paramedic who had been admitted to her floor, a guy who had driven across the country to come help out in New York, a guy with a walrus mustache who she thought must be a tough motherfucker to rock that thing in the Bronx. She knew about the legions of out-of-towners coming to help, some of whom wound up in her borough looking like they'd just come out of an Oz tornado, blinking with "Where am I?" confusion. But she knew the virus came for tough motherfuckers too. And if he was coming into the ICU, no one knew which way his illness was going to go.

The Chef

Made with Love

May 31–November 3, 2020

THE NIGHT A FELLOW Louisville chef was shot down in his own kitchen, Nikkia was staying cozy with family. The last few days in May were bringing a new onslaught of strife to her city, and this time it seemed best to avoid it. George Floyd was murdered in Minneapolis on the 25th; three days later, the Louisville *Courier-Journal* published audio of the anguished 911 call Breonna Taylor's boyfriend placed moments after she was shot, in which he wailed her name and sobbed: "Somebody kicked in the door and shot my girlfriend!" The protests that followed that weekend devolved into looting and vandalism, the governor sent in the National Guard, and the mayor imposed a 9:00 p.m. curfew.

Nikkia spent Sunday evening chatting with her family about the protests, about Breonna Taylor and George Floyd, about how strange it was for the city to impose a curfew on grown adults, about why the National Guard was in the streets. Just the week before, gun-toting pro–Second Amendment demonstrators had marched outside the governor's mansion, shouting opposition to coronavirus restrictions and then hanging the governor in effigy from a tree outside the state capitol, to the tune of "God Bless the U.S.A." The chest of the stuffed effigy was emblazoned with caps-lock motto "SIC SEMPER TYRANNIS"—"thus always to tyrants," the Latin phrase John Wilkes Booth uttered after he shot President Abraham Lincoln in the head. Nikkia wondered why these protesters hadn't warranted a National Guard response. It didn't look like a coincidence to her that they were being called out amid racial-justice protests instead, and if the point was to stop the looting, why was the looting still happening?

She was about to head home from her aunt's place around midnight when her sister looked at her phone and said someone had been killed on 26th and Broadway, far from the downtown protests, in the city's predominantly Black West End. A chef, it turned out—a man who shared Nikkia's love for food as a way to bring people together and give back, who was known to offer free meals from his modest barbecue shop to struggling neighbors and police officers alike, a small-business owner trying to make it through Covid. He'd served for three years as a chef at the Volunteers for America Kitchen, where, as a kid, Nikkia used to go help out with her mother.

David McAtee's was another life that bent toward giving and then was violently taken away.

Nikkia learned more about him the next day from testimonials to Chef David posted on Facebook. The takeout barbecue stand he had operated on a busy corner of town was called YaYa's BBQ, for David "YaYa" McAtee's Rastafarian name. He lived in a basement apartment with a kitchen on the first floor and a few grills outside, and he served hot dogs, sausages, hamburgers, and ribs from a blue canopy tent at the end of the driveway. He was planning to buy the lot, maybe in a year or two, but in the meantime he'd built up a joyful small business feeding a piece of the city that didn't have a lot of good food options—West Louisville was what the sociologists called a "food desert," where it was easy enough to find fast food and liquor stores but difficult to get quality meals or healthy groceries. If a customer couldn't afford a plate of his grilled meat in homemade sauce, David wouldn't charge.

YaYa's intersection was a weekend hangout spot for the neighborhood, where friends would listen to music in the parking lot outside Dino's Food Mart and could go get some of David's barbecue across the street. That Sunday night into Monday morning, the curfew passed and people stayed out, and a few hours later, police and National Guard units moved in to disperse them. When officers started firing pepper balls, people scattered and pushed into David's kitchen while he stood at the door. Within minutes, a bullet struck him in the chest, killing him. He was 53.

The police later said that David shot at them; surveillance video from inside his store shows him twice leaning out and raising his arm before being hit. His nephew Marvin, who was in the room at the time, told the *Courier-Journal* that he and David thought they were about to be looted by the crowd of strangers rushing into the store; they didn't at first realize the shots they heard were from pepper balls, and as the shooters moved closer to David's kitchen, at least one struck near David's niece, who was standing beside him. Nor did they realize that the source was law enforcement, whom Marvin said his uncle would never target. In fact, Marvin told reporters, some of the cops who hung out at YaYa's had advised David to get a gun to protect himself from looters, days before David himself was shot.

David's death and its aftermath convinced Nikkia and Lindsey that they had to get their kitchen started as fast as they could. Their mission had become even more of a necessity for Louisville, particularly the West End, where more than a hundred mourners gathered outside YaYa's the day after its proprietor's death, sharing their grief and anger, while the body that had once been David lay for hours in the street. In the afternoon, the crowd on the pavement stood silently, fists raised, while one short, sturdy bald woman unrolled a forlornly hopeful rendition of the hymn "Amazing Grace."

Then that night around 1:00 a.m., looters broke into the Kroger grocery store two blocks from where David had been killed, raiding the pharmacy as well as the beer and baby-product aisles. The store shuttered itself temporarily, knocking out one of the few places to get fresh food and medication in West Louisville. That Kroger was one of three full-service grocery stores for the area's roughly 60,000 people spread across nine neighborhoods. West Louisville residents were also among the least likely to have access to cars, so a trip to the grocery store could take multiple bus rides and much of a day. The difficulty of accessing fresh, healthy food options had contributed to poor health conditions in that segment of the city even before the pandemic. By one estimate, living in West Louisville could shear 15 years off a person's life expectancy. Residents lived an average of 67 years, compared to 82 on the other side of town.

Many people had difficulty enough trying to feed themselves

and their families as employment evaporated under the state's Covid restrictions. In March and April, the first months of pandemic shutdowns, the Louisville metropolitan area had lost more than a hundred thousand jobs, and the unemployment rate had blasted past 16 percent—landing Louisville among the top 10 worst-hit cities in the country for pandemic job losses, along with tourism and manufacturing centers such as Las Vegas and Detroit. More people were relying on government assistance to buy food, and now, many in West Louisville had nowhere to go to buy it, just as they were getting their benefits at the beginning of the month.

Even then, Nikkia observed, the community stepped up. Within hours, Kroger's West End neighbors had come out to help sweep up the glass on the parking lot.

It also didn't escape Nikkia's notice that the National Guard had been blocks away from the store that night. Its members had managed to disperse a crowd at a gas station and kill David in the process, but they hadn't prevented the looting they'd been called out to stop.

■ ■ ■

Nikkia and Lindsey masked up and met up the following week at one of Edward Lee's restaurants, 610 Magnolia in Old Louisville, where Lindsey had served as the general manager. Edward was there, and a few others who had worked on the restaurant relief project, who could help to coordinate donations for food and funding. They sketched out a schedule—250 meals, packaged for families of four, three times a week—and a distribution plan. They pondered staffing, and Nikkia, eager to lift up a new generation of chefs and anxious to make up for lost classroom instruction, started working on her plan to recruit some of her culinary students.

As for space to cook in, among the pandemic's deserted restaurants was Milkwood, the very restaurant that had launched Nikkia into her culinary career only five years before. It was no longer serving its adobo fried chicken and specialty brown-liquor cocktails. No one was there to admire the tasteful exposed brick.

Edward announced on Facebook that after seven years, he was closing Milkwood. "I want to help my community of Louisville," he wrote. Of Nikkia, he went on: "This is no longer my kitchen. It belongs to her. We are not here simply to feed those in need. We are here to inspire the next generation of Black chefs in Louisville through pride in our professionalism, passion and integrity."

The place was located downtown, just six blocks east of the so-called 9th Street Divide that stood as an informal barrier between the West End and the more prosperous parts of the city, and Nikkia wanted to make sure the food would be accessible to the communities they wanted to serve. She and the others ultimately settled on three drop-off locations where volunteers could hand out meals to whoever wanted them: Two community centers in the West End and a now-closed bar in the Smoketown neighborhood, where she had grown up—another food desert that had just lost a grocery store.

Lindsey spent a week securing funding and stitching together food sources. Many people and organizations wanted to help. A food bank, Dare to Care, would provide the bulk of their ingredients. Maker's Mark, one of Kentucky's famed bourbon distilleries, would supply potatoes and squash. A farm-focused nonprofit, the Berry Center, would come through with a weekly veal delivery worth thousands of dollars.

The person Nikkia was especially touched to hear from was Ruth Moore. She had taught Nikkia at Western High School and was undergoing cancer treatment in April of 2020 when she began to experience Covid symptoms. That was the beginning of an ordeal that would condemn her to a hospital for 43 days, 27 of them spent on a ventilator. Her recovery was so unlikely that it made the news, a rare feel-good story of the pandemic. Friends, neighbors, and family greeted her homecoming with a line of about 50 cars, and well-wishers honked and held up signs to greet her. Shortly after that, and having learned of Nikkia's new venture, she offered her former student extra squash from her garden.

Nikkia, who had only recently been a mere peeler of fava beans and assembler of salads in Milkwood's kitchen, would now claim the space as hers to run, which meant having to get enough staff in place as quickly as possible to assemble thousands of meals a week. Meanwhile, she hadn't set foot in this kitchen since 2016, and it looked roughly the same except for the disappearance of the big ice-cream machine—which is to say, it was all wrong. Milkwood had been a stylish *a la carte* joint, abandoned abruptly a few months before, evidence of the last dinner rush still visible and small plates and sauté pans everywhere, all of it useless. She was not running a hipster tapas place but an industrial-scale feeding operation in a pandemic. She needed big pots and spaced-out workstations and protective equipment.

She spent the next week deep cleaning and transforming the space, while she looked for her new chefs. She found them in her virtual classroom, three recent graduates and one current student, and started hunting down funding for their salaries. As it happened, Louisville's mayor was set to plow about a million more dollars into the city's SummerWorks youth-employment program, on the strength of big new donations from local organizations concerned at the city's economic and racial strife—and, Nikkia suspected, in part out of guilt over the city's violence and its handling of protests. Eventually she'd get her student employees paid $10 an hour for 30 hours a week, to help them support themselves and their families while they worked to support others' families, too.

By Friday, June 12, Nikkia and the others were ready to formally kick off their new venture. They celebrated with a small cookout at YaYa's BBQ Shack, where they resuscitated the grills and the take-out tent in celebration of David McAtee's life. A local Black-owned restaurant, Sweet Peaches, provided side dishes, and Nikkia raced around serving up burgers as David's old neighbors, friends, and family members shared memories over free plates of food. Then, on Monday, June 15, two weeks after David's death, Nikkia opened up her community kitchen in his name.

David couldn't feed people anymore. But McAtee Community Kitchen would.

■   ■   ■

A week at McAtee Community Kitchen looked, typically, like this: On Monday, a colleague would go to the Dare to Care food bank and report back to Nikkia what was on offer that day. The two would place a massive order—300 pounds of fajita meat, anyone?— and get it hauled back with a borrowed truck from a philanthropic farm outside Louisville. Churchill Downs offered extra freezer space. Nikkia and her students would back-engineer a menu from the haul, and Nikkia, ever mindful of David McAtee, made sure to include at least one barbecue option per week. Then they'd pack up the meals for ease of popping in the oven and truck them over to the drop-off points to be ready to hand out between 4:00 and 6:00 p.m. on Mondays, Wednesdays, and Fridays. Volunteers in protective gear at each location would hand out the food to whoever showed up needing it, till the meals ran out.

For their first meal they made chicken legs, rubbed with brown sugar, chili powder, garlic, and onion, then smoked, with a zucchini-and-squash vinaigrette pasta salad on the side.

It was hell.

It *sounded* tasty, but chicken legs didn't really fit in the nine-inch round aluminum serving pans they had, and the bones made closing the flimsy cardboard lids nearly impossible. The original transportation plan, of packing six pans apiece on sheet pans and then stacking them up in the delivery van, proved a disastrous mess as the pans kept sliding around, strewing chicken thighs all over the back of the van.

Resolved to avoid bone-in meats and sheet pans in the future, Nikkia's team next tried putting trays in boxes stacked on top of each other, only to find that the weight of the boxes crushed the lids on the pans below so that food squished out and mashed potatoes covered the sides. Trial and a lot of error eventually brought them to a transportation strategy involving insulated bags and cardboard dividers, which made for tedious packing but generally intact meals arriving at their drop points.

The kitchen itself would at times thwart the cooks in it. It featured only one oven that could fit six trays, which meant staff had to stay alert and rotate the food in and out frequently. If one of her students forgot to weigh out portions or did the math incorrectly, they could run out of food while dozens of meal trays still sat empty, necessitating a scramble of reapportionment to ensure enough meals.

The initial idea had been to run the kitchen through August, to see Louisville through a difficult summer, but as fall approached demand wasn't letting up. Nikkia determined to just keep cooking until someone told her to stop. Meanwhile, a grand jury decided on September 23 that the police officers involved in the raid on Breonna Taylor's apartment would not be charged with killing her, returning one "wanton endangerment" charge against an officer for also firing on a neighboring apartment. Protesters poured into downtown Louisville and blocked off the kitchen altogether; two police officers were shot and injured in the demonstrations. That, despite everything else, was the first time the community kitchen missed a food delivery.

She knew what it meant to keep making these meals. She mostly stayed in the kitchen, but on occasional visits to the drop-off points she'd seen some of the folks who depended on her. There were homeless people who opened and ate the cold trays right on the sidewalk. There was a set of parents with children who arrived all jammed onto a motorcycle, which appeared to be their only mode of transportation. There was a family in a middle class–looking car, who didn't appear to be in such dire straits, but maybe needed help to get through the week. The volunteers weren't going to ask about income level; if one of their meals could help remove a source of worry even for a night, that was success.

At Trouble Bar in Smoketown—named in tribute to the civil-rights activist and congressman, John Lewis, who had urged Americans to "get in good trouble" to redeem the country's soul—the owners organized a books and toys drive for kids in addition to handing out meals. Two grandmas became regulars, picking up books and meals and chatting with volunteers about their grand-kids, then returning the books the following week and taking new ones as if the bar was a library. At the California Community Center in the West End, an elderly neighborhood man named Charles came to get food and sit on the steps for the company, talking about his love for Diana Ross.

Handing out meals and coordinating volunteers there, Scotty Hauser, who had spent decades in the music industry prior to the pandemic, loved to hang out with Charles, and loved to watch the way people helped out their neighbors even if they were struggling themselves. He struck up a friendship with a man who would pick up multiple meals to deliver to people he thought might need the food. Like Scotty, the man had lost his mom before the pandemic; they bonded in shared grief, two motherless sons. And then one day the man showed up with something of his own to give Scotty: his mom's old *Better Homes and Gardens* cookbook. The man had had no way of knowing that Scotty had grown up on the cookbook in his own house or that, to Scotty, the gesture meant everything in the world.

Nikkia's own favorite memory was of two men getting out of a truck, and one asking the other why they were stopping at this place in particular for food. "Because," she heard him say, "I know this food is made with love."

■   ■   ■

It was supposed to be a just a routine test, the quick kind you could get in a parking lot, with a Walgreens staffer sliding a swab through a crack in your car window so you could swab yourself and return the results in a little sealed bottle. She wasn't feeling bad, but she was trying to be responsible, because she was planning a cautious trip out of town to attend a spaced-out wedding. It was going to be Halloween themed and she'd already made costumes for herself and her boyfriend—Roger Rabbit and Jessica, except that she was Roger and he was J., wearing a red tuxedo instead of a red dress.

Nikkia got a call with the results a few hours later and learned that her travel plans were shot. The test was positive.

She felt nothing. Nothing Covid-related anyway, though she did feel fear, and anguish that she was going to miss her friend's wedding. The kitchen had a batch of meals hours away from delivery, and it was a pre-Halloween menu the team was especially proud of: meatloaf with mashed potatoes, individually wrapped cups of candy, and, now that they'd hit their stride to the point they could make their own desserts, homemade cookies. People were counting on these meals to show up on time, she knew. But if the test was right, would feeding them mean putting all those people at risk of getting sick? Was she really stuck between possibly infecting people and letting them go hungry?

She shut herself up at home and called the kitchen's manager. She hadn't handled the food herself, but she'd been in the building the day before, sitting 10 feet away from colleagues in the dining room as they planned their menus for the next week. What if she had infected her own students, who had just showed up to help the community?

The staff shut down the kitchen and dispersed to get everyone tested. Trays of meatloaf formerly bound for the hungry and the struggling went into the garbage instead. All the meals the staff had begun to prep for the remainder of the week were trashed too. This was a precaution, and Nikkia felt sick about it. She feared Covid. But if this was a false positive, all that food was going to waste for no reason.

Her contacts' test results started filtering back. Soon it was clear that no one else in Nikkia's orbit—not the kitchen staff, not her boyfriend, not her mom—had tested positive for the virus. Another rapid test she herself took came back negative; the person who called to deliver the results to Nikkia speculated, of the positive test result delivered just days before, that maybe Nikkia had been sick and the test had caught the tail end of it. Or maybe this was some-thing else entirely. Rapid tests, designed to detect chunks of viral protein, could deliver false positives as well as false negatives—they could mistake some other bodily protein for a Covid trace or alter-natively miss actual bits of the virus altogether. The more-precise polymerase chain reaction, or PCR, tests actually hunted for yet tinier genetic traces of the virus, though, as the name suggested, they also required sophisticated lab analysis to deliver results, which could take days. So Nikkia arranged a PCR test, her third and most invasive test in a week—the kind where a health worker in PPE jabs a swab up your nose, past the point it feels like it should stop. Then she waited, and hoped. If all went well, this could just be a temporary setback. The kitchen staff could lie low for a few days and then go back to work if Nikkia's test, like all the others, came back negative.

It wasn't just those who needed the meals who counted on her, but those who made them. The kitchen staff was relying on her for a paycheck in the pandemic.

She was still waiting on the results when someone from the state department of health called her.

This was part of Kentucky's attempt at contact tracing, a virus-containment tool that had been part of the most successful campaigns against Covid in other countries. South Korea, for instance, was famous for its aggressive "test-and-trace" program, which had enabled the country to locate the virus with precision, isolate those exposed, and avoid nationwide lockdowns in favor of targeted containment. The United States had largely left contact-tracing efforts to state health departments, which had pursued it with varying degrees of enthusiasm. Some states had pretty much given up, because the sheer profusion of cases, and the days-long delays in returning test results to many patients, made the technique effectively useless: Tracers just couldn't trace enough people.

But a tracer had found Nikkia, albeit two full days after her positive test, and with no knowledge of the intervening two tests. Those tests, a Kentucky Department of Health staffer told her, wouldn't change what her government was now asking her to do: stay home, isolate. Two weeks.

Nikkia didn't know if the kitchen would survive that.

PART THREE

PART THREE

The Patient

Waking Up

March 28–August 31, 2020

Huy was running around town, kicking ass, fighting crime. He was some kind of superhero, but he was a bit frustrated he wasn't one of the really cool ones like Iron Man. He was, instead, a D-list superhero like Ant-Man, but nevertheless he was on the side of righteousness and had strange abilities and defeated bad guys. It was quite fun, a very nice change of pace from a Facebook desk job. Certainly better than being in the hospital, sedated and breathing through a tube.

Which is where he actually was, unbeknownst to him, undergoing all kinds of tests and subject to constant observation. His dreams had taken him out of that nightmare and elsewhere, into adventure instead.

And the days passed and passed. The Ant-Man continued to right wrongs.

On March 31, Huy spent his 36th birthday unconscious with a tube down his throat. The one-day death toll from the virus reached its highest point yet in the United States as 811 were reported to have lost their lives, bringing the total death toll in the country above 3,800. Some hospitals were intubating so many patients that they were running out of sedatives.

His mom turned 64, on a ventilator like her son, on April 3. Daily death tallies had continued to climb and set a new record that day as 1,224 people reportedly perished, breaking the previous record set only the day before. "Flatten the curve" was the public-health man-tra, and one of the president's coronavirus advisers, Deborah Birx, told Americans from the White House to try to avoid even going to pharmacies or the grocery store for the succeeding two weeks.

In that period, Huy's sister quarantined herself from her hus-band and child in Nevada, got hospitalized and then discharged. His dad cleaned the empty house in Milpitas day after day and awaited updates on two different loved ones from two different hospitals.

And the Covid death toll in the United States more than dou-bled between Huy's birthday and his mom's, to more than 8,000, with 60,000 dead worldwide.

■   ■   ■

Huy's fever had fallen, and his breathing seemed to be improving. His doctors started to lower the dosage of the medication keeping him under. Ant-Man retired at some point, and Huy's conscious-ness returned, barely, to his hospital room, where he became aware that there was something in his mouth and wondered what the hell it was, checking it out with his tongue. It was extremely uncomfort-able and he had no idea why it was there. With his eyes still closed he put his hands onto whatever it was and tugged.

He ripped the breathing tube out of his throat.

Satisfied he'd taken care of the weird thing in his mouth, he went back to sleep.

■   ■   ■

Huy floated upward slowly, semi-submerged in sleep, until he finally broke the surface of consciousness again and the hospital room seeped into his vision. He looked around. A name was written in black marker on one of the windows facing out into the hallway. "Taylor Swift." *Huh?* Sleep tugged him back under before he had much time to think about her, or the unembarrassed Tay fandom he'd harbored ever since her country-to-pop evolution in her third album "Speak Now." Then he drifted up again, blinking back into the world and the weird scrawls on the window. More names. "Death Cab for Cutie." "Ed Sheeran." *Why?* More confusion. *Wait a minute, I like these bands.*

He found out later that a social worker assigned to his case, to help keep his family informed and keep him comfortable, had asked his sister for ideas. In an effort, maybe, to deliver some familiarity to his dreams or remind him of the great world waiting for him to wake up to, they had tried to ensure that his favorite music was played as he slept.

He wished he could remember the music, to be able to say to his sister that Taylor Swift had led him toward the light. But he couldn't remember much of anything.

He had come unfastened from time, didn't much know or care if he was awake for hours or days, which offered only fragments of events in any case. He saw doctors in the room, and someone asked him to say his name and wiggle his toes. He discovered he could do both. Someone asked him what day it was, which irritated him, because how the hell was he supposed to know what day it was? He could offer the year, 2020. Okay then, what month? March, he guessed. He knew he'd checked into the hospital in March. He was surprised to learn it was already April. So it was a good thing he'd paid his bills.

Days or minutes passed, he couldn't be sure; he drifted out, drifted back, people in protective gear swam into view and faded away. At some point he tried to FaceTime with his family but typed in the wrong passcode too many times and locked himself out of his phone. He hallucinated. He slept. He did not eat. A feeding tube kept him sustained.

He woke again startled to see his sister. She was staring at him through the screen of a laptop that Nghề had dropped off at the front desk to be taken into the room so the family could communicate now that Huy's phone wasn't working.

"Oh, hey," he murmured. His vocal chords were feeble from disuse and the abuse of the breathing tube. He saw something move in the frame that held her face. "What's that?"

"That's your nephew."

He was still drugged up and barely capable of holding a conversation. She spared him, for now, from what she knew.

Keeping in touch through the laptop proved complicated. Huy's sister kept asking him to leave it open; Huy kept forgetting and then having to try typing in the password his dad had stuck to the computer on a Post-it, which he couldn't do because his motor skills were too impaired even to let him type, so a nurse or another hospital staff member would have to keep letting him back in. But it was through the laptop that he finally learned what had happened to his mother while he was out.

It was during another disembodied, non-bedside conversation, with his sister, largely recovered from her own illness, unable to deliver the crushing news in person. "You need to know," she told her brother, "mom's not going to make it." The ventilator was not going to save her; there was bleeding in her brain, and despite the machine that was keeping her lungs working, her body could shut down at any time.

His sister's face floated on the screen. Huy was still wrapped in post-coma fog, getting more lucid, but even so this was barely possible to absorb. It seemed to him the family had just been convincing her she'd be all right on the ventilator, and she was just bitching about her doctors giving conflicting advice. Wasn't that just a few days ago? Hadn't he himself only been under, running around as Ant-Man, for like three days?

"It's been 16 days," his sister said.

He was trying to fit reality back together and now it was getting smashed again. He had seen his mother walk herself into the hospital, and she wasn't coming out alive. He'd known it was a possibility—she'd had what people now called "underlying conditions," including a minor heart attack the previous year—and yet it also didn't seem possible. Hopelessness overtook confusion and forced tears out of his eyes and sobs out of his throat.

They cried together. But they did, potentially, have one comfort that would be denied to thousands of other families in the same miserable position. Mothers, fathers, sons, daughters, were dying of

the disease alone for fear of its horrible contagion. Nurses and doctors were holding up cell phones for family members to say goodbye
without ever being able to hold a hand or sweep the sweaty hair off
a forehead. Huy and his sister were grieving through their screens
right now as many others had through the pandemic, but Huy was
going to survive. And his whole family had already had Covid,
which meant that the ICU doctors at his mom's hospital were willing to make an exception and let them in, to be next to Liên when
she was taken off life support. Nobody really knew whether the
virus could infect someone twice, but the risk seemed manageable.

There was just one catch, his sister explained: Huy, who couldn't
even coordinate his fingers to type in a password or lift food to his
own mouth, let alone walk, needed to get himself well enough to get
out of Stanford hospital as soon as he possibly could.

To get released, Huy would need to prove to his doctors that he
could feed himself independently. He'd have to be able to respond
to questions to his doctors' satisfaction, start learning how to walk
again, and generally demonstrate that he could be all right outside of the hospital. Newly grieving and barely coherent, he faced
the most important project of his life, and the deadline was cruelly
tight. If he missed it, he'd lose the chance to see his mom one last
time and say goodbye.

He called for a nurse. He was ravenously thirsty, but also not
allowed to have water because of the risk he'd choke. The nurses
would bring him ice chips with a spoon, and he was to hold a chip in
his mouth and wait for it to melt. He decided to use the opportunity
to teach himself how to eat again.

He was surprised at how difficult it was, how quickly the most basic life skills—or in his mom's case, life itself—could disappear. His hands shook as he lifted the spoon. He missed his mouth; he bonked his nose. He kept working. When he managed with great effort to get his hands to work and guide the ice onto his tongue, he told himself to focus and not just let the ice melt there. The next step was to get his mouth to work, moving the ice around inside, trying to chew.

Then there was the problem of his legs, which had similarly atrophied. His doctors at first wouldn't even let him swing his legs over the side of the bed. He liked keeping his mattress at an angle, but kept sliding down, and rather than allow the doctors to scoot him back into position he insisted on doing it himself, pulling himself with his arms using one of the bed handles, while his legs lay there unhelpfully.

He tried lifting them, moving each to the left and to the right, stretching his toes to make sure he could feel them. He thought it would help to keep trying to stimulate the muscles, and that this should prepare him to take his first steps. Finally came physical therapy, half-hour sessions in which two therapists would bring in a walker, and guide him to sit up, pivot to the side with his legs dangling off the mattress edge, lean his hands onto the walker, try to put his weight on his feet, and slowly stand up.

That was when he realized getting out of the hospital was going to be much harder than he'd thought. He couldn't support his own weight.

Over the course of multiple sessions that day and the next, though, his feet eventually learned again to stabilize him, and his legs held him up. He learned to sit, and stand himself back

up, and sit, and stand himself back up. Next he learned to shuffle his feet and get used to the sensation of shifting weight. And
then, finally, forward movement. A therapist told him to push
the walker forward a few inches, and then step forward to meet
it. Then to do it again. And again. Until he could lurch slowly
around the hospital room.

By the first evening that he knew of his mom's condition, he
had slipped into project-management mode for his own health,
sketching out next day's tasks and trying to locate who was responsible for getting them done. He learned that he needed to eat not
just one but two meals before he could be discharged, and he put
in his breakfast and lunch orders at the same time, insisting that
lunch be queued up and brought out as soon as it was ready. He
found out which nurse would then remove his feeding tube and
asked to see her. He inquired about her work schedule and told her
to make sure to be around at lunchtime, because he wanted the
tube out immediately after that.

He went to sleep determined that, though he'd spent the whole
day eating ice cubes, he was going to feed himself a real breakfast
and lunch, and then escape.

His dad and sister waited in the car while Huy waited on his
tube removal, then waited some more as hospital workers gathered
his belongings and pulled a wheelchair into his room. Finally, on
April 16, at around 4:00 p.m., Huy was wheeled out the door of
Stanford's hospital to make the journey down the peninsula to see
his mother alive one last time.

Alongside his dad and sister, he watched as doctors decreased
her oxygen and increased her medication. Right before she took her

final breath, he asked to be wheeled out of the room. He couldn't bear to see it.

Afterward, one of her doctors gave Huy's family a bag of Liên's stuff and offered condolences. And that was it. They left.

■   ■   ■

Liên was the sort of person who, had she died at any other time, would have had the kind of well-attended funeral that closes out a life well-lived by a person well-loved. She had practiced her Buddhism in service to others, including, once she'd gone into real estate, helping some monks find the property to open up a new temple. For many years after that, she had devoted substantial time and money to cooking meals there, feeding people after regular services or when they came to their own family funerals. She'd make Huy go with her on grocery and supply runs for the temple, and if Huy sometimes did this grudgingly, Liên was determined to provide support and to try to help people feel better. Even if people skipped the prayer parts of Sunday services and just showed up for the free food—she wasn't there to question anyone's intentions.

Covid restrictions limited her funeral to no more than 10 people. Monks from Liên's temple showed up in full PPE, chanting over her. Huy was grieving and weak and angry at the world, but was nevertheless struck by the reverence the monks showed his mother because, typically, it was the monks themselves who were revered and bowed to. Now he saw them bowing to her.

The monks kept chanting through the service and alongside Liên's casket as it was wheeled out of the room and into the crematorium. She was never alone, right up to the moment her body turned to ashes.

Over the weeks that followed, Huy relearned how to walk, recovered his strength, returned to remote work, and became preoccupied with how to assist others afflicted with his former illness. The government was pouring millions into ads pleading with survivors to donate their blood plasma, the yellow liquid that would otherwise be carrying red and white blood cells around in the donor's body. The substance was also a storage bin for the Covid-fighting antibodies that had already helped the donor defeat the disease, so doctors saw potential to put them to work in other sick bodies. If a given store of plasma had helped one person to survive, maybe it could help others. Clinics were already trying this out experimentally, and early data from tens of thousands of patients seemed to show the treatment could improve a Covid patient's chances of survival.

Huy signed up for an appointment at the Red Cross and, on the arranged day, sank into one in a row of recliner-like chairs to let a machine slurp his blood, pull out the plasma with a centrifuge, and return the remainder, now a chilly liquid pouring back into his body. It was a long process, about two hours, and he passed the time watching *Ant-Man* on his phone until he noticed the centrifuge stuttering, spinning up and slowing down. Red Cross workers came and fiddled with the machine but no one could fix it. In the end Huy could only complete half a donation.

He came back a few weeks later to donate again. He completed the other half of the donation before the machine broke again. By then some scientists were cautioning that it wasn't clear how well convalescent plasma treatment worked for Covid patients, anyway.

With the machine mishaps and the scientific uncertainty, Huy had done the plasma-donor equivalent of taking home an A-minus to his tough-to-please immigrant parents. But at least there was a chance his plasma could help someone, maybe even save somebody else's mom.

And, thinking about what his own mom might be doing now if she could, he had another idea.

He knew his family wasn't the only one grieving. He also knew that, without his mom, the temple she'd served for so long was missing a healing presence at a time of enormous uncertainty and pain. The temple could not hold Sunday services anymore, and funerals were restricted. But the monks there still wanted to give away meals to the bereaved, and Huy had recovered his strength enough to reprise his role as errand boy at the temple again, even without his mom roping him into it. So that's what he did.

He liked to think his mom would approve. He'd tried to do his part.

The Paramedic

Procession

April 19–October 27, 2020

BEFORE HE WOUND UP in Michelle's ICU, Paul, too, was trying to do his part—had been trying for decades, and here in New York had been trying for almost three weeks by the middle of April. He wanted to do even more. But it was getting more difficult. Paul was back from the medical trailer and by his rig when Jerrod Estes returned from the food trucks near the start of that night's shift on April 19 and asked how he was feeling. Paul confessed, not too hot.

This sounded like a significant admission, a semi-stoic mini-complaint betraying something seriously wrong. Jerrod knew from his years in emergency services that anytime a cop, EMT, paramedic, or fireman told you they didn't feel well, it meant they really didn't feel well, particularly if that person was an older man. That, given the circumstances, was probably worth a trip to the hospital, and Jerrod tried to point this out to Paul, who got stubborn, wanted to stay and work, and *really* didn't want the fuss of getting trucked out on one of his team's own ambulances. Jerrod vowed discretion;

they'd get Paul in the back of his truck and just very casually roll out of the lot after alerting Incident Command what they were up to. Paul relented.

They ended up in a nearby emergency room with nothing to do but wait. Paul seemed more worried than anything else that Jerrod insisted on hanging out there with him—if Paul couldn't work right now, certainly someone had to. But Paul didn't have any family in New York, and Jerrod didn't want to leave him alone. He spent eight hours chatting by his side. In the end, the hospital discharged him to rest back at the Sheraton. That's where he stayed, fighting for breath. Personnel from the zoo would leave food outside the door, and colleagues would talk to him through it. Paul stayed stoic as his health declined.

Montefiore took him in soon after. He was once again on the wrong side of the ambulance, pulling into the dim driveway that led underground into the hospital's emergency department, patient not paramedic. He'd sat down here with colleagues at times during the deployment, as it was one of the refueling stops in addition to being a hard-hit hospital. Familiar sight, strange city.

This was the kind of scene he knew from other people's worst days—a place you could mistake for a normal parking garage, if not for the ambulances and the bustling people in medical gear, opening to a sickly yellow-lit corridor that emptied into a large room, curtain-separated beds lined up against the outer walls, one section crammed to overflowing with coughing, suffering people, nurses in a middle bullpen manning monitors, everyone grim and efficient.

He felt sick but resolute, almost as if Paul Cary the paramedic had sufficiently reassured Paul Cary the ER patient that he need not worry. Speaking to the ER residents on duty was difficult but not impossible; he managed to describe what had brought him to New York in the first place, and declare he was determined to get better and get back out there. At that point much of the Colorado crew had completed their deployments and gone home, and he was one of only four left in New York. Though Paul stayed on, of course he missed his family. So he had to get better soon to see them, too.

The doctors took chest X-rays and confirmed what was already clear: The fog had crept over his lungs on both sides. He was instructed to roll over onto his stomach, a technique called proning that helped some patients reduce the pressure on their lungs. It was uncomfortable to hold that position for hours, but Paul didn't resist. He was used to giving instructions and resigned to its being his turn to follow them.

He texted his Colorado friends, Alissa and Royce and a few others, that he had Covid. He asked them: If you're praying people, pray for me.

■   ■   ■

In Colorado, Chris had been keeping tabs on his dad, talking or texting every few days. Just days before he found out Paul was in the hospital, they'd been discussing who would pick Paul up from the airport when he got home. Chris didn't know that Paul had changed his mind and decided to stay.

Nor did he know right away when his dad started to show Covid symptoms. Paul wasn't about to call and start people worrying.

The call Chris got from the Bronx on April 21 wasn't from his dad, and it wasn't about arranging an airport pickup. It was from Montefiore Medical Center, and it was about arranging medical care.

Paul was still conscious and fighting when Chris reached him on the phone that day. But he was breathing as if hiking up a mountain. And when Chris called the day after that, he sounded more like he was running up a mountain. By then, Paul had decided to go on a ventilator, and Chris had a feeling this talk might be their last. But he didn't really know what to say.

Chris was in regular touch with Paul's doctors, who at first sounded encouraging; Paul was at least stable. But days went by. Paul's kidneys began to fail. He started on dialysis. The longer he remained unconscious the clearer it became that he wasn't going to wake up. Chris's brother, Sean, had lived and worked overseas for years, and his mom and dad's marriage was over. It was going to be up to Chris to take his dad off life support.

Chris wasn't planning to go be there; no one was asking him to. Paul would by no means be the first or the last to die in the pandemic without a loved one near him. But at the last minute Chris decided he needed to see his dad one last time. It was easy enough to find room on a flight. Chris took a largely empty plane to LaGuardia on a Thursday, April 30, where a police escort was waiting to take him to the hospital. When he reached Montefiore's ICU, there wasn't much of a goodbye to say. It was already too late; his dad wasn't really in that body pierced by all those tubes. Chris wasn't even allowed to enter the room to sit next to him; he looked through the glass of the ICU window at his father breathing one last time before medical personnel turned off the ventilator. Chris had seen his grandmother removed from life support years before, and remembered it taking about a week for her to die. But his dad was gone almost immediately. No gasping for air, no resistance.

Paul wasn't going to get to hear "Empire State of Mind" to accompany his journey out of the hospital.

Instead, friends loaded him back into an ambulance to take him to the funeral home. Royce, who had returned to Colorado before being called back to cover Paul's shift, was now deputized as a pall-bearer for the friend he'd made just a few weeks before.

■   ■   ■

When the ambulance pulled away from Montefiore and made its way down the street, Royce could barely believe what he was see-ing. It was late on Thursday, the rain was pouring not just down but sideways in a vengeful April wind. Royce had until then been inside the hospital, getting instructions from New York firefighters on the proper way to drape a flag over a coffin, absorbed in the absurdly tedious logistics of death. He wasn't prepared for the crowds of ambulances, fire trucks, and cop cars lining the streets nearby, almost an impromptu streetside funeral, following the radio alert announcing Paul's death. Signal 5-5-5-5: death in the line of duty.

The trip to the Bedell-Pizzo Funeral Home in Staten Island, which sat about six blocks from a fire station near the southern tip of the island and had hosted many a remembrance for the city's fire-men, was about 40 miles, and took an hour and 40 minutes. Chris rode shotgun in his father's old ambulance, and he could quickly see that the gathering for his dad wasn't just a hospital-neighborhood affair. All along the route, he looked out at lined-up emergency vehicles, their red, amber, and blue lights leaving smears of color on the glistening pavement. At points on the way, people stood outside the trucks in their coveralls, getting pelted by the rain just to watch Paul go by. Finally, Royce and the other pallbearers carried his coffin past another line of saluting firefighters and into the funeral home. A kilted bagpiper stood under one of the scrawny trees outside and offered a soundtrack to the line of light-blue Ambulnz trucks, a tiny flag flying from one of its pipes.

Then another drive halfway back the way they'd come, to the airport in Newark, New Jersey, where on the tarmac Chris was greeted with more of the same, more salutes, more cameras, more reporters, bagpipes playing "Amazing Grace." He tried to avoid attention, and chatted with some nurses who, like Paul, had volunteered to deploy from Colorado to the harder-hit East Coast. One had even taken a class from Paul. Royce helped to carry the flag-draped coffin into the waiting airplane. Then Paul was on his way home.

A similar scene awaited him when he returned to the community he'd served all those years before New York called, where he'd expected to return in order to keep serving. Instead, Paul came home to lines of fire trucks, lights flashing along the highway, medical workers outside The Medical Center of Aurora in the cool night in their scrubs and masks, some holding signs, "TMCA HEARTS PAUL." EMTs and paramedics saluted, standing outside their trucks. Friends and neighbors lined other sidewalks, holding candles, holding flags, holding signs. "ALL GAVE SOME, SOME GAVE ALL."

∎   ∎   ∎

Paul was buried in the Olinger Hampden Cemetery in Denver, his grave distinguished by a simple plastic marker. A few months after his return, a former colleague named April Johnson started a GoFundMe to raise the $8,000 necessary for a proper headstone, inscribed with a poem by a Wichita fireman named A. W. "Smokey" Linn, who wrote it in 1958. Like Paul, Smokey was a compulsive fireman, who according to family legend ran into a burning barn when he was 15 to save his grandfather's Model T truck parked inside. He somehow came out with the seat of his pants smoking, his granddaughter said in a speech after he died. His poem, since christened the "Fireman's Prayer" and featured on fire-station walls and Web sites and wall hangings around the country, started out as an appeal to God he wrote after being unable to rescue children from an apartment fire. The words that would mark another firefighter's grave more than 60 years later testified to the value of trying despite knowing you couldn't save everybody—not even yourself.

> *When I am called to duty God*
> *Whenever flames may rage*
> *Give me the strength to save some life*
> *Whatever be its age.*
> *Help me to embrace a little child,*
> *Before it's too late,*
> *Or some older person*
> *From the horror of that fate.*
> *Enable me to be alert*
> *And hear the weakest shout*
> *And quickly and effectively*

To put the fire out.
I want to fill my calling
And give the best in me
To guard my neighbor
And protect his property.
And if according to your will
I have to lose my life
Please bless with your protecting hand
My children and my wife.

The CEO

The Stockpile

June 7–August 31, 2020

Paul's ventilator hadn't saved him. In fact, as Michelle knew well and Huy's family had learned in Liên's devastating loss, once a patient was sick enough to need such a machine, that person's survival was very much in question. And yet, if a patient truly needed a ventilator and couldn't access one, there was little question that patient would die. Chris's operation in Kokomo churned on into the summer, everyone hoping their machines would beat the odds for the desperately sick and offer a gateway to getting well again.

By June, the Ventec–GM venture was still new and sprawling, some parts still barely sticking together as if with string and chewing gum. It depended on remarkable individual dedication to meet weekly production deadlines that were ramping up from the hundreds into the thousands as the venture raced to deliver 30,000 ventilators by August 31, under the terms of a government contract. There was Joe Cipollone, the engineering

VP, whose wife back in Washington received a cancer diagnosis within weeks of his move to Kokomo but reassured him she'd be fine. There was Debby Hollis, a GM worker who thought of her elderly mother as she signed up to switch from manufacturing circuit boards to ventilators, knowing that her mom, or people just like her, might need one.

And then there was Reggie Hopwood, the pilot whose job, in the absence of reliable commercial cargo service due to the pandemic, began to involve personally flying circuit boards from Washington State to Kokomo in one of his own small planes.

Somewhat incongruously for a man from southern Missouri who had once killed a grizzly bear in Alaska, Reggie had a *Seinfeld* quote for nearly every occasion ("And *you* want to be *my* Latex salesman . . ."). He worked for a small subcontractor of GM's, a freight-on-demand company called McNeely Charter Service based in West Memphis, Arkansas, and at 58 had spent his entire professional life in the aviation business, from the time he was 18. Normally McNeely moved a lot of auto parts around, but with vehicle manufacture shut down or diminished, there wasn't much freight to move. McNeely was busy instead with one of its niche operations, which was ferrying day-old baby chickens to farms. It was Reggie who'd spotted postings to bid on circuit-board deliveries, and Reggie who'd signed up for a handful of trips, each a three-day ordeal of getting to Washington, getting the required rest between flights, then getting to Kokomo and back to West Memphis.

He flew deliveries at night in order to bring the materials to the factory in time for the morning shift. But on the morning of June 7, he wasn't there.

People were already at the factory, anxious to start their shifts, aware they didn't have time to waste but watching it slip away regardless. And then the news filtered through the floor that the pilot wasn't coming.

He had been on his way from Washington, in a twin-engine Mitsubishi cargo plane, when weather conditions diverted him from a planned refueling stop in Huron, South Dakota. At 1:40 a.m., he'd landed instead in Sioux Falls, South Dakota, where he fueled up and got going around 4:26 a.m. The plane was still climbing when the right wing started to dip, rolling the plane over and then pulling the nose down. It crashed shortly after takeoff, killing Reggie. The pandemic delayed an investigation, preventing officials from the National Transportation Safety Board from traveling to the site to collect evidence.

Chris Kiple had been on a flight of his own with Chris Brooks, on their way back to Kokomo from Washington, when Reggie's plane went down. They got the news in a phone call from a shaken colleague after landing in Chicago, while they were securing a rental car for the three-hour drive south. Kiple tried to absorb what had just happened, the sacrifice involved in this operation and how it was asking so much of so many people already—and now a life had been lost in its service. He didn't know Reggie Hopwood or the family, including two adored grandkids, he had left behind. He did know that the news would be an emotional blow for the team, and he also couldn't help worrying about the next deadline bearing down. His colleague was now telling him that absent this circuit-board shipment, they weren't going to make it. The team was building so quickly on such a compressed timeline that they were constantly falling behind and catching up and falling behind, losing 12 hours here and making it up there. They needed to get the supplier to ready a new shipment as quickly as possible, before they lost another day, and then they'd be back to scrambling to try to regain lost ground. Kiple felt the force of simultaneous pressure and heartache for Reggie's loss.

Both he and Brooks recognized that their job remained what it had been: trying to save as many lives as possible. They could barely stop to mourn the dead. They got into the car and drove to Kokomo.

■   ■   ■

The team pushed on, through tragedy and illness, through logistical snares and personal traumas, and the ventilators still rolled off the line and into UPS trucks to hospitals and to struggling patients' bedsides. And even so, a disturbing number of Covid patients died while intubated. Some doctors had looked at the springtime death rates and grown doubtful that ventilator use would even help the most severely ill patients. In some cases, it could even harm them. Early in April, right around the time the Kokomo plant was opening, small studies in China and the United Kingdom had found that most Covid patients didn't survive ventilation—the worst statistics came from Wuhan, where of one set of 22 patients that got on ventilators, only three got off alive. Another study of patients in New York hospitals published later the same month found that close to 90 percent of 320 ventilated patients whose fates they could account for did not survive.

The disease was doing things to the lungs that doctors had never seen before. Health-care workers were witnessing patients with "happy hypoxia"—whose blood oxygen levels plummeted even as they were able to speak normally and avoid gasping for breath. Respiratory ailments often made the lungs grow stiff or filled them with fluid, making breathing difficult and impairing the flow of oxygen into the blood. But some Covid patients seemed to be breathing comfortably and losing oxygen anyway, almost as if the very air they were breathing just didn't have enough of it, like the air at the top of a mountain. No one could figure out why.

This led some doctors to question whether ventilation was really the appropriate procedure for many Covid patients or whether in fact they were treating a brand-new disease following old procedures and damaging patients' lungs in the process. For a pneumonia patient with stiff lungs that couldn't inflate properly, it might make sense to use a ventilator to force air in—the way you'd have to blow harder to inflate a balloon made with particularly thick rubber. But if the lungs weren't really resisting air intake, you might apply way too much pressure and pop the balloon.

As the pandemic evolved, however, so did treatments and knowledge of what the sickest patients needed. Easing pressures on some hospitals that had faced the earliest brunt of the pandemic, for instance those in New York, left institutions better able to allocate staff with the appropriate expertise to operate and monitor the machines. Montefiore's critical-care medicine chief attested that among ventilated Covid patients, "we win more than we lose." Other hospitals elsewhere in the country had found Covid ventilator fatality rates closer to 20 or 30 percent. Newly deployed drug therapies such as remdesivir and dexamethasone were aiding the chances of survival.

And fears of widespread ventilator shortages calmed by the end of the summer. Early eye-popping estimates of need had turned out, so far, to be wildly off the mark. This was partly because the scariest models of the early days had overstated the disease's spread and severity, partly because public-health measures such as social distancing and masks had reduced the spread, and partly because treatment for the most severe cases had evolved. Doctors, spooked by ventilator survival rates, were trying other forms of treatment, putting off intubation as long as possible or avoiding it altogether. At the University of Chicago Medical Center, for instance, physicians were pursuing ways to "prevent the vent," such as with high-flow nasal cannulas, which they found to help patients avoid intubation in dozens of cases—though cannulas did put caregivers themselves at more risk, because the cannulas could blow aerosolized virus into the air.

Elsewhere in Chicago, at Weiss, Suzanne Pham had also found she could wait longer to intubate patients than initial guidance had suggested or avoid it by using oxygen therapy and close monitoring. Yet the machines remained a critical last resort for the sickest patients, and with the hospital's fortified stockpile of ventilators, she never again had to contemplate the horrible choices she'd have to make if the supply ran out.

By July, Ventec and other companies in the United States had churned out 100,000 ventilators, and the headlines had changed from worries about a shortage to the reality of a surplus. One frightening spring estimate that had popped up regularly in March news reports, for example, suggested that given its existing supply, the United States could be short more than 700,000 ventilators needed to help Covid patients. But by mid-August the Department of Health and Human Services had deployed about 15,000 ventilators to aid states around the country and had added more than 94,000 to the federal stockpile, and the federal government and some state governments were canceling orders for the machines. The president was vowing to send some of the excess overseas.

Chris wasn't sanguine about the numbers, however. To him the lesson of the prior few months was just how quickly the system could get overwhelmed, and as he watched the disease's spread accelerate again heading into the fall, and saw the exponential spikes in the numbers, he had a sinking feeling. The expanded federal stockpile of ventilators was a good thing to have, not just because of this pandemic, but because this one wouldn't be the last. But you also had to be able to deploy a ventilator to the right place at the time it was needed, and man it with the appropriate expertise. Difficult as it had been to ramp up production of ventilators so quickly, you couldn't manufacture new respiratory therapists in a matter of months. Still less new hospitals to put them in—Kokomo could churn out ventilators, but 16 counties in its own state of Indiana didn't even have a hospital. The end of summer was bringing a surge of new Covid cases into the Midwest, and a pandemic that had begun for Americans on the coasts, then attacked the South and West, continued to conquer new geographies. It was no longer meaningful to talk about Covid hot spots: The entire country was a hot spot.

■   ■   ■

One hot and sticky August evening, Chris was in the basement of the Kokomo factory at a reunion of sorts. The leadership teams of the Ventec–GM venture were all together for the first time in months, having converged to see the last of the federal government's 30,000-ventilator order ship out the door. The Kokomo plant would keep going, filling orders from states and hospitals, as Covid case numbers and demand for the machines remained high around the country. But the team had reached a milestone, and a partnership that hadn't existed six months before had pulled together and achieved something resembling a miracle.

They swapped war stories as they waited for the last machines of the federal order to come off the line. They looked tired; some had thickened from stress and overwork. But they also seemed awestruck by what they, and so many who had been working long factory hours in Kokomo, had accomplished. Ventec had ramped up ventilator production approximately 80-fold since March and was now churning out a new machine every seven minutes. The prior week had been exceptionally difficult, in the way that many, many other weeks had been exceptionally difficult, as team members tracked down parts from around the country and scrambled to get them in place on time. Just as they'd had for many weeks before, they had a deadline racing at them, and it was never quite clear until the last minute that they could actually meet it. They'd all been living just on the edge of failure for so long, and now, maybe, they'd taken a few steps back toward safety.

This time they seemed to be in good shape. Their final machines were boxed up and ready to go; they had to be out for delivery by August 31, and here they were, set to get boxes to the loading dock well before midnight. Chris signed the last box with a blue Sharpie. "Amazing team effort," he wrote. "This has truly been an example of what can be done when people work together to solve the impossible."

Chris watched as a tractor trailer pulled into the loading dock to haul the boxes away. Or tried to. Minutes drained away from the remaining time before Ventec's last deadline while the driver tried to navigate the dock's tight corners and aggressive angles, steering one way and then another, backing up, moving forward. Chris stood there with his GM and Ventec colleagues, including Chris Brooks and Joe Cipollone, all exhausted and eager to claim victory, while the world's most interminable parking job just kept going on in front of their eyes, for 15 minutes, then 30, then 45. He began to wonder seriously whether this would be the thing that forced them to miss their final and most important deadline. Others discussed who should hop in the cab and take over or whether they should get a pallet jack and try to move the boxes out to the truck themselves rather than waiting for the driver to get to the loading dock. They were just about to achieve what they'd thought impossible, and yet the simplest thing was becoming the most difficult. Thwarted by parking. Of course.

Ultimately it took nearly 15 of the top minds at GM and Ventec to help steer the truck into the loading dock, where it rested and took up its lifesaving cargo.

Everyone clapped and cheered.

Such a motley cast of actors had come together to make this whole thing possible: wildly different private companies; federal, state, and local officials; engineers and truckers; even, at the very beginning, a random assortment of philanthropists with a hashtag and a hope to #stopthespread. The bitter truth was that the spread hadn't stopped and wasn't about to. Chris Kiple had seen a team get focused on a single mission and move mountains, but the Covid mountain had stayed stubbornly put. He'd seen people push past the limits of human endurance, together, and he'd also seen human limitations cruelly enforced, from a too-tight parking spot and even unto death.

The Chef

Keep Going

NIKKIA ALSO REACHED a milestone, but it wasn't one to celebrate. The McAtee Community Kitchen was initially only
supposed to operate through the summer. Instead they'd made it up
to the beginning of November. Then one little nasal swab changed
everything.

Winter was starting, and Covid cases were spiking, and the
McAtee kitchen was a small one. Even though two subsequent tests
likely proved Nikkia's first result to have been a false positive, Lindsey, who had helped found the kitchen and now managed much of
the financial and logistical operation that kept it running, feared
for the safety of the staff and the volunteers. Maybe they'd escaped
infection this time, but maybe it was only a matter of time before
their luck ran out.

And only a matter of time before their funding ran out,
too. Donations were wearing thin so many months into the pan-

demic, rent for the old Milkwood space was a significant expense, and the kitchen staff had just thrown out a week's worth of food.

Lindsey felt she had no choice. McAtee Community Kitchen had to close.

When she called to tell Nikkia, her chef's overwhelming feeling was guilt. Nikkia had only done what she was supposed to do in taking the stupid test in the first place. Now people were going to go hungry because she'd done the right thing.

Nearly a year into the pandemic, this virus was still wrecking lives and plans even where it hadn't actually infected someone. Healthy people were still staying home by the millions as a precaution. More and faster Covid tests across the country were supposed to help people live and work more safely by identifying who was sick and should isolate. But the FDA had warned that rapid tests could give false positives, and the agency couldn't pinpoint just how likely this was. Even more worryingly and more frequently, tests could also give false negatives, at a rate that varied from test to test and study to study but could be up to 30 or even 40 percent. Such results could trick sick people into believing they were healthy enough to be in contact with others when in fact they were spreading the virus and might need treatment.

It fell to Nikkia to break the news to her students that not only were they not going to be serving thrice-weekly meals to their neighbors in need any longer, but those who had worked alongside her for so many months to stand up and staff this place, to learn and to give back, were out of a job. So were the three adult staff members, some of them with kids, and one of whom had already been laid off when the pandemic hit earlier in the year, and who would now be forced to scramble to find something else and make Christmas happen.

Nikkia couldn't help thinking that if she hadn't taken that first test, none of this would have happened. And she didn't really know what to hope for—that she'd actually had Covid, making shutting down the right thing to do? Or that, as she strongly suspected, she'd gotten a false positive and had never been sick—and thrown good food away, and friends and colleagues out of work, for nothing?

She told Lindsey she felt like a failure.

But Lindsey had already been helping to cook up something much bigger while Nikkia was running the community kitchen. Within a week after it closed, the Lee Initiative created a new employment and relief program designed to feed Louisville and reach even more people. As Nikkia prepared to head back into the classroom after winter holidays, her friends were working with her public school system to use the schools as distribution points for family meals. Jefferson County Public Schools had kept trying to provide meals through the pandemic for the many students who relied on their free lunches, but those meals did little to address the hunger engulfing their families. Nor did they help to address the ongoing unemployment crisis wracking the city and the country, particularly in the hospitality industry.

So the Lee Initiative launched a new partnership, with Nikkia's school system and Churchill Downs, among others, to hire 50 out-of-work chefs and set them back to cooking, in the racetrack's unused kitchens. They were doing a scaled-up version of Nikkia's operation: this time they'd offer 8,000 meals a week for families of four, to be distributed for twice-a-week pickup at different schools. This had begun to take shape in August, around when the community kitchen was first expected to shut down, but it had taken months to realize. It finally came together right as Nikkia's venture was shutting down, and as a difficult winter including a Covid surge and new business closures bore down on Louisville. Once again the ethos was, if not to save the world entire, at least to feed some families, ease their hunger, and save some worry for working parents struggling to pay bills and educate their children at home.

Nikkia was prepared to come cook if she got the call, but was otherwise looking to the future. She planned for a relaunch of her kitchen in 2021, this time with elements of Chef Edward Lee's Youth Hospitality Program, which had helped kickstart her own career as a chef. She wanted to build on the success of recruiting students, and maybe even expand beyond Iroquois, her own school, so that the community kitchen could serve meals while it served as a training ground for a new generation of chefs—Black chefs in particular, she hoped. She wanted to expose them to different styles of food service through two of Chef Lee's restaurants—fine dining at 610 Magnolia and whiskey-and-burger style at Whiskey Dry—while still offering free weekly meals to the needy in the name of Chef McAtee.

She was taking a bet on hope over uncertainty. With research ranking bars and restaurants high among many culprits for Covid spread, the Kentucky governor had careened between different sets of restrictions for months, experimenting with changing capacity limits and curfews and then, at the end of November, shutting down indoor dining altogether for more than three weeks. Nationwide, some 10,000 restaurants closed temporarily or permanently over the course of the fall, taking another 18,000 jobs with them. It was hard to see in the depths of a Covid winter, with her own kitchen shut down, but she had to believe that someday this all would end, and that she could prepare her students to seize that much brighter future, whenever it came. Someday there would be real graduations, followed by real graduation dinners at packed restaurants where the tables creaked under too many plates of barbecue and succotash, and the bourbon flowed for the grownups. But she wasn't going to just wait for that future. She was going to help build it.

She was also struck by the compassion of her Louisville neighbors as Christmas neared. One organization, Change Today, Change Tomorrow, launched a "Bless the Block" campaign, through which individuals and businesses could donate money to specific blocks in the West End, to fund meals and Christmas wish lists for the families there. The same organization had also, since early June, provided free groceries to the West End food desert through the #FeedtheWest program, and its leader, Shauntrice Martin, planned to open a Black-owned grocery store soon to improve food access in that part of the city. Louisville could be a violent, segregated, and unjust place. But Nikkia knew that most of its residents didn't want to see people suffer, and many tried to fix it.

To her, there was a simple lesson to draw from the year's setbacks and struggle and chaos, its ever-receding hopes for healing, its relentless interlocking plagues of disease and injustice and violence. In November, Travis Nagdy, a young protest leader in Louisville locally famous for his huge hair and his bullhorn, was shot in an apparent carjacking as the city smashed its annual homicide record. He'd told the Louisville *Courier-Journal* only a month before his death that he found purpose in the movement to seek justice for Breonna Taylor, and that as a self-described ex-foster kid and felon with no GED, he'd been close to suicide until he found something to fight for. Once again people poured into the streets to mourn and protest, and many adopted his motto: *Keep going.* It was this that Nikkia kept telling herself as a difficult year trudged to its conclusion.

It was still hard, and the light was still months away, and restaurants were still dying, and West Louisville was still underserved, and yet—what else was there to do? "That's what we all have to do," Nikkia said. "I think that this year has amplified for me what I've always thought of when you are met with tragedy, and hurdles in life, and struggles, and just adverse experiences, is that you can feel it, and it can hurt, and you can feel how you feel about these things. You can feel upset about Covid. You can feel upset about Breonna Taylor being killed. You can feel heartbroken about David McAtee being killed in his kitchen. But at the end of the day, what are you going to do about it?

"You've got to let it light a fire under you at some point and do something about it. You've got to keep going. You can't let tragedy and you can't let all the people who have died this year—you can't let their lives go in vain.

"You've got to keep going, because you're lucky enough to still be here."

The Nurse

Organizing

April 30, 2020–February 3, 2021

Mᴉᴄʜᴇʟʟᴇ'ꜱ ᴠᴇʀꜱɪᴏɴ ᴏꜰ "keep going" was: "You get knocked down, you get sick, you get traumatized—you get the fuck back up." Just like Paul Cary, she was used to losing more than she won and still showing up to play. But some of the losses were harder than others, and the loss of Paul, whom she'd cared for and even been able to speak to before he went on the ventilator, was one of them. She had cried on the April day when she found out he was going to die. She knew by the ICU monitors what was coming. In other units, you might be in a room with a patient without knowing whether that person was asleep or dead, but ICU patients were so closely observed, with their vital statistics on display at the nurses' station, that their fates were visible from down the hallway. So she knew it when the sturdy-seeming dude who'd traveled across the country to help wasn't going to make it.

He would keep a piece of her heart for what he had done for the city.

But around the same time, and very slowly, the ICU beds started to free up. Michelle noticed one day that a single bed was unoccupied in her unit, after so long operating at and beyond full capacity, and figured that filling back up was only a matter of time. But as May crept forward, more and more ICU beds stayed empty.

On May 29, for the first time since the pandemic started, the Montefiore hospital system reported no deaths at all.

■   ■   ■

The worst of it seemed to be over, for now. Michelle went on union leave days later, on June 1, changing her main focus from patients to the nurses caring for them, trying to help fix some of the problems she was convinced had killed people during the pandemic. Her main preoccupation was staffing, and she worried in particular about a sister hospital, Montefiore New Rochelle, just to the northeast in Westchester County.

New Rochelle had been one of the country's early Covid hot spots, and an incubator of the kind of drastic public-health measures that would soon cascade across the country. It seemed almost quaint, after months of lockdowns and reopenings, that on March 10, the city's cluster of 108 known coronavirus cases had been possibly the largest in the United States, double the known number in New York City—though in hindsight it was clear the virus had been circulating much more widely, undetected by tests. The New Rochelle outbreak, thought to have originated with a lawyer who attended services at a local synagogue, prompted the governor to take what then seemed like a radical step: imposing a "containment zone" within a mile radius of the synagogue in question, in which schools and large gathering places (including synagogues, churches, and community centers) had to shut down for two weeks, while other businesses (including restaurants) remained open, and the National Guard delivered food to the homebound. New Rochelle had also pioneered New York's first drive-through testing centers, borrowing from South Korea's aggressive testing strategy to contain the virus.

By December the city was once again a microcosm for much of the country, with its cautious summer reopening followed by a creeping Covid resurgence. This time, the virus spread appeared tied not to large gatherings, but to smaller get-togethers in people's homes. Hospitalizations were edging back up, too, and although Montefiore administrators said their hospitals now had 90-day stockpiles of PPE, nurses reported still having to reuse N95 masks too often and fearing that the hospital in New Rochelle—a community facility that cared even for patients who couldn't pay—wasn't ready for the wave of Covid cases everyone could see was coming. Already a nurse and a nursing assistant had died of COVID-19 there.

Michelle had a new fight on her hands as she thrust herself into contract negotiations in New Rochelle. The nurses had been negotiating for about two years, and everyone had stopped haggling for a few months because of Covid while they focused on simple survival—their patients' and their own. But as the wave of emergency receded, nurses were picking through the wreckage and trauma it had left behind. Management was happy to call them "heroes" until it came to annual pay raises, in which case the bosses felt entitled to take 3 percent per year and the front-liners should be happy with 2. Everyone kept thanking them for risking their lives for their patients, but God forbid anyone heed them when they begged for more staff to help them. They shouldn't *have* to risk so much just to barely afford living in New York, while the Montefiore CEO pulled in more than $10 million a year.

Michelle felt like she had been saying it forever: People died when nurses were overwhelmed. Everyone knew this—it was well documented, in country after country, that as nursing patient load increased, so did the risk to the patients. "Safe staffing" wasn't just a nurses' union crusade, either; hospitals and politicians, including New York's governor, had raised alarms for years before Covid about nursing shortages. But what was anybody doing to get new ones? Hospitals around the country were saying they didn't have enough nurses, they didn't have enough doctors. Not enough, not enough. Michelle knew what it was like to sit with the grief of losing a patient and wonder if she could have saved him, if only she'd had more time. What was the plan to fix it?

In the spring, Cuomo had begged retired and out-of-state nurses to help, but this wasn't a sustainable strategy in the long term. By the end of November, Cuomo was back to fretting about shortages as statewide Covid hospitalizations quadrupled from their summer lull of 900 a day, except that the out-of-state cavalry that had helped save New York in the spring—with some 30,000 health-care workers like Paul Cary charging into the state to help—wasn't coming this time. This time, the rest of the country had its own problems to deal with. Hospitals in Texas and Utah were openly discussing rationing care.

Clearly the country wasn't going to fix a long-standing shortage in less than a year, in the middle of a pandemic. In the long term,

Michelle thought there were just too many barriers to getting the necessary education; she felt lucky to have been able to take out loans for her degree, though now she felt like she was on a hamster wheel of debt seven years later, even though she had no kids and lived with her family. But in the short term, there had been ample time to at least spend the few months' reprieve training existing nurses to take on ICU care, so that when the new surge came, hospitals weren't putting yet more patients at risk with nurses unused to the complications of critically ill patients. No such luck there, either.

New Rochelle's nurses had resumed contract negotiations over the summer, which were conducted remotely and digitally now. Michelle was scornful of this, too. If the hospital was, as its leaders insisted, doing everything it could to protect the nurses, why did they feel the need to protect *themselves* from the nurses? Wasn't that an admission that those nurses were indeed shouldering the risk of infection? Michelle spent her time behind the scenes polling her colleagues. Are you okay with a 2 percent raise a year? With or without retiree health? Do you think we should fight for this? What do you think the next steps should be?

She thought the nurses at New Rochelle were timid, and that they needed some Michelle love. Some were having to hustle among eight patients apiece. "You guys need to go to the Bronx," she'd say, "because in the Bronx we don't play that shit." The union there had fought to set a maximum of five patients each for med-surge nurses, though Michelle bitterly observed that the hospital didn't adhere to that, anyway.

On Thanksgiving, contract negotiations were continuing to go nowhere, and Michelle was home with her family watching the pandemic-lite Macy's parade—crowds discouraged, route reduced, and much of it pre-taped—when the ad came on. It opened with nighttime New York scenes: a bridge and skyscrapers and a crosswalk, glimpses of a traumatized city still uncharacteristically subdued. Then it showed musicians tuning up on the street or on fire escapes. Michelle slowly recognized a scene she'd only heard about from someone at her Bronx hospital. While New Rochelle nurses were getting ready to strike, one day the staff at Montefiore Moses had gotten a shift-change serenade from what amounted to a street orchestra of dozens. And now, in the television ad, the orchestral strains of Natalie Merchant's "Kind & Generous"—the one with all the "thank you"s—were playing over shots of surprised and moved health-care workers stepping out of the hospital.

"To the healthcare heroes saving New York," proclaimed the text on the screen, "Montefiore thanks you."

Michelle lost her shit.

"Just fucking shoot me," she burst out. Jaws around the room hinged open: an aunt, an uncle, and her little brother had come over even though Michelle had been hesitant about the tiny crowd, which was still a major break from her usual habit, in previous years, of inviting basically anybody to come stop by. She was furious. How much did all this shit cost? How many thousands of dollars did it require to broadcast two minutes of this propaganda during Thanksgiving-parade prime time, when her friends were still worried about running out of protective gear? "I feel real appreciated," she spat. "Whole lot of fucking bullshit, that's what that smells like."

She was tired of the "hero" shit. Truthfully she'd always found it enraging. Most days she didn't feel brave or even particularly useful—for all she knew people had died in the spring because she couldn't handle her patient load. Much worse, every time she saw that word, she saw a sickening excuse, a way for negligent leaders to hide from their failures and persuade themselves that they were doing right by the ones, like her, cleaning up their messes without enough support.

Don't call me a fucking hero, she wanted to scream. To her, "hero" wasn't a term of individual honor, it was a sign of national shame. You didn't see people in Australia or Taiwan going on about their health-care heroes. Because they weren't overwhelmed and dying. Because people in power had bothered to plan, protect them, and fucking deal with the virus.

She was tired of being thanked. She didn't need thanks. Nurses needed help.

Meanwhile, Montefiore New Rochelle gave its final, take-it-or-leave-it offer, including a better wage increase still shy of 3 percent, funding for the union pension fund, and no mention of staffing levels. In response, almost every single one of the hospital's 200 nurses voted to go on strike.

They marched for two days in the cold outside the hospital. They hoisted signs about safe staffing and told reporters about their fears for the inbound Covid surge. Management accused the nurses of abandoning their patients and trying to dictate staffing assignments. When the strike ended, some nurses found their expected shifts canceled: The hospital had transferred some patients to another facility and said it didn't have enough patients to warrant a full staff. Nurses accused the hospital of locking them out of their jobs.

In the end, the tussle resolved nothing. The nurses eventually returned to work, contract negotiations stayed deadlocked, and the Covid patients kept coming.

■   ■   ■

For all that, Michelle was happy on Christmas. She got her dad a blanket to commemorate the family dog, Tank, who had died in February, and was extremely pleased with herself to make such a tough guy cry. Her grandma, who loved dressing up with jewelry ("like she's a long-lost queen of Spain or some shit," Michelle joked), got a $300 bracelet, which soon wound up on the floor. Grandma had fallen a lot this year, gotten kicked out of the house to wait out the family Covid outbreak, celebrated her 90th birthday with just her immediate family after everyone had recovered, and finally here she was at Christmas.

Michelle looked around. It had been a terrible year. She'd had no way of knowing, in Tank's awful last moments, when a vet had come to the house to put him down because the family knew he would freak out if they actually took him to an animal hospital, that losing this beloved family member wasn't going to be the worst of it, that she'd come so close to losing her parents, too. For all her anger and determination to keep fighting the hospital system, she took a moment to simply feel grateful to have her family around her and still alive. She'd held the hands and spoken to the families of enough dying people to know exactly how important that was. Whatever else was happening, whatever power she was fighting, her family was alive and together. And happy.

The hospital, of course, was never far away. Union leave would end at the beginning of February. She worried that even though she was technically among those slated to get a vaccine first—the CDC had recommended that health-care workers and residents of long-term care facilities get the first doses, followed by "frontline essential workers" and those over 75, and then other groups moving down the level of risk—there were already signs of shortages, just as there had been with protective equipment. She'd heard of administrators getting shots before frontline health workers, though the hospital said it had offered the vaccines to front-liners immediately after the shot was authorized. She half suspected she wouldn't be vaccinated by the time she had to go back to caring for patients.

Plus, she was nervous about the vaccine itself, and understood why others were, too. She felt like almost every authority figure of the pandemic had lied to her in one way or another, and now they expected her to trust them on a vaccine? She was nervous about the new genetic technology being used. But she told herself she had to trust the science. She'd heard that a Russian vaccine used a more traditional method, but then again, apparently the Russians who took it were told not to drink for six weeks, so maybe Americans had the better end of the stick.

In the meantime, she was thinking about Florence Nightingale, the activist English nurse of the nineteenth century, who had tended to wounded Crimean War soldiers, used statistics to convince lawmakers of the importance of sanitation, and pushed for better care for the poor. That showed Michelle what nurses could accomplish, and she was determined to make her own change. She'd spent the past year watching nurses do impossible things.

"Those of us who pushed through those few months," she said

in December, "I'm grateful for us because that resiliency reminded me that we're going to be all right.

"It's going to get worse. Shit's going to hit the fan again. But even then, we're going to be all right."

She got her first Pfizer vaccine shot on January 8, and the next one three weeks later. In February she was back with patients, with reason to hope for a better year.

The Vaccine Developer

Emergency Use

MICHELLE GOT HER VACCINE less than a year after the coronavirus's genetic sequence had first appeared online and set off a competitive hunt for an inoculation. Hamilton's team at Moderna was the first on the trail. They had identified and finalized the genetic sequence for their vaccine candidate within two days after seeing the virus's genome. They'd gotten their first batch ready for human testing within 25 days and then, following preliminary tests and FDA approval, their partners at NIAID had gotten it injected into the first human arm within 63 days, making theirs the first Covid vaccine candidate to be tested in humans. By the time Operation Warp Speed showed up in May, they were already within days of reporting good interim results for Phase I trials.

All of this had happened in record time, and the team just kept running as fast as it could. By the end of May, on the strength of their deal with BARDA, Moderna had been able to start its own second, larger phase of the trials, which would involve hundreds of participants—half of them in the high-risk age cohort over 55—and would compare the vaccine's performance against a placebo. Simultaneously they were designing the final, crucial phase of the trial, to measure the shot's efficacy in thousands of volunteers prepared to risk the side effects of an unknown drug for a chance to help get the world out of the pandemic.

That was the trial that would show, once and for all, whether the vaccine worked. The plan was to recruit more than 30,000 volunteers from at least a hundred sites all over the country; inject half with the vaccine and half with the placebo, with neither the trial's participants nor its scientific investigators knowing which person got which; and then wait to see who got infected with the coronavirus as they went about their daily lives. When enough participants got sick, an independent panel would compare how many of them had received the placebo shot versus the actual vaccine. Fewer sicknesses among the vaccine-takers than among those who'd been given the placebo could mean the vaccine was providing some protection.

By early July, with the pandemic fully in its summer surge and Covid infections rising in 39 states, with more than 130,000 Americans dead of the disease, the team was just about ready to launch the biggest clinical trial of the company's history on the fastest timeline any company had yet attempted.

But then, suddenly, the momentum stalled.

Moderna hadn't hit a medical snag or a manufacturing problem. The FDA, the National Institutes of Health, and Moderna's own review committee had already approved the trial protocol, the plan for how Moderna would inject and monitor its human volunteers. Hamilton thought everyone who needed to sign off had signed off. But as Moncef had warned early on, the thing about government funding was that it also came with government input.

Moncef should know: He'd had to resign his position at Moderna after being tapped to lead Operation Warp Speed.

Now, with the trial's start date of early July bearing down, Operation Warp Speed wanted to reopen debates over data collection and monitoring that Hamilton thought had been settled in May, before Operation Warp Speed had even existed. The new regime came bearing new principles for all its private partners to observe in clinical trials, for the sake of comparing results across different vaccines. All perhaps reasonable in the abstract, but Hamilton was incredulous to be hearing about it now. Where were these principles months ago when Hamilton and her team had been bleeding themselves dry designing a clinical trial for 30,000 people? And where were they when the FDA had signed off? And why, when Moderna was so far ahead of all the other companies under the Warp Speed umbrella, was her company now being asked to slow down, allowing everyone else to catch up?

Hamilton lost weeks debating and adjusting, only to fall further behind the exploding pandemic, as the virus spread from its early epicenters on the East Coast to besiege states in the South and West. July set a new record for case counts in the United States: 3 million cumulatively, and then 4 million just 15 days later. She watched as the date she'd planned to start the next phase of lifesaving research came and passed. Another 20,000 people in America died that month, pushing the national death toll over

150,000, and the Kaiser Family Foundation estimated that 36 states, accounting for more than 70 percent of the U.S. population, were now "hot spots."

By the time Moderna was permitted to begin its final trials on July 27, Pfizer, one of its chief competitors, which was also building an mRNA vaccine in partnership with the German company BioNTech, had caught up. Pfizer was a pharmaceutical juggernaut with $52 billion in annual revenues—Moderna's haul was $60 million in 2019—and its leaders had judged that accepting Warp Speed help in the research phase wasn't worth the trouble, though they did get a near $2 billion contract to sell doses once developed. In Hamilton's best-case scenario, despite Moderna's frantic early start, the company would trail Pfizer in collecting data. Both vaccines involved two injections, but Pfizer's were spaced three weeks apart, and Moderna's took four. This meant that no matter what, Moderna would be at least a week behind.

■   ■   ■

Hamilton also had to consider, as trial sites prepared to open up and enroll participants, how to ensure that the population of volunteers reflected the diversity of the country at large. Those sites were going to enroll as many people as they could as quickly as they could—it was a pandemic, and besides, they got paid by the participant, so there was moral and monetary incentive to move quickly. But Hamilton knew from conversations with academics and vaccine advocacy groups that there would come a time, given the political moment in the country, the protests and the wrenching racial-justice debates and the fact of the virus's disproportionate decimation of Black and brown people's lives, that Moderna would have to prove its study actually represented the people getting sick.

Yet that same political moment, in which police brutality had intensified minority communities' fear and distrust of the state, made it all the more difficult to generate trust for an experimental, government-funded vaccine. Only about 32 percent of Black adults reported themselves likely to get a vaccine, according to one poll by the Pew Research Center, versus 52 percent of white adults. Vaccine developers and trial investigators faced a racial Catch-22. Black people and other minorities were bearing the brunt of illnesses and fatalities from COVID-19. They were disproportionately likely to be working in essential jobs that put them into close contact with other people all the time, in grocery stores, public transportation, health-care facilities. To end the pandemic, those at highest risk should be the highest priority for a vaccine, and a trial would have to prove it worked for them. Given concerns among experts and the public about the speed of vaccine development and Trump's own attempts to influence the timing, this just looked like the country was asking Black people and other minorities to shoulder a new set of risks to make the country safe.

It wouldn't be the first time. A medical experiment on Black men in Tuskegee, Alabama, beginning in the 1930s left hundreds of them untreated for syphilis for decades, just to watch the natural progression of the disease, even after penicillin was proven to be an effective cure in the 1940s. The study only shut down after the Associated Press exposed it in 1972. A later study from the National Bureau of Economic Research found that Black men exhibited more mistrust of the medical system than did other demographic groups, and that this contributed to lowering the group's average life expectancy. Beginning in the 1950s, doctors treating a young Black woman named Henrietta Lacks took cell samples from her and shared them with researchers without her consent; after her death from cervical cancer at age 31, her cells "became a workhorse of biological research," as *Nature* put it, while her family reaped no compensation from the profits companies made off her. The so-called HeLa cell line, in fact, facilitated cancer research, the development of *in vitro* fertilization—and, nearly 70 years after her death, research on COVID-19. By infecting HeLa cells with the new coronavirus, scientists were able to observe the way it attacked human cells, helping inform how a vaccine could stop it.

And just as vaccine researchers and experts in the United States were fretting about achieving diversity in clinical trials for a COVID-19 vaccine, two French doctors showed on television why the legacy of such events endured. They were discussing whether a tuberculosis vaccine could be effective against Covid. "Shouldn't we be doing this study in Africa, where there are no masks, no treatments, no resuscitation?" one of them mused. "You are right," agreed the other.

Hamilton was regularly reviewing demographic data about who was participating in the trials. By August it was clear that they were overwhelmingly white. Once again Moderna's leadership, and Hamilton, faced the agonizing prospect of slowing down, in an effort to recruit a more diverse trial population. And once again, they pumped the brakes, this time to encourage clinical sites to work harder on outreach and education in minority communities. In the end, they raised minority participation from 24 to 37 percent in the space of a few weeks.

This was a success for experimental design, but it still didn't mean that, assuming the shot became available, most Americans would actually take it. Polls conducted in June and August of 2020 found that anywhere from a third to half of Americans weren't sure they'd get a Covid vaccine. One found that bipartisan supermajorities worried "the vaccine approval process is being driven more by politics than by science." Americans' skepticism only grew as the months passed and the trials continued; by September, according to the Pew Research Center, the number of people reporting they'd get a vaccine had dropped by 21 percent since May, from 72 to 51 percent. Nearly 80 percent of Americans worried the process was moving too fast.

This was a centuries-old skepticism with a new twist. The first vaccine, developed by Edward Jenner in 1796 in England, was an inoculation against smallpox that involved exposing people to the related, but less lethal, disease of cowpox. Doubters at the time worried that sticking "a bestial humour into the human frame" would end up producing cow-like features in children: ox-y faces and patches of cows' hair on the body. It also didn't help that the very first recorded vaccination was viscerally icky—a scratch with a darning needle dipped in infected cow pus. Nearly 160 years later, Dr. Jonas Salk's 1950s-era polio vaccine helped deliver the United States from a recurring epidemic that, in its peak year in 1952, killed 3,000 people and left 21,000 paralyzed. Within six years of the vaccine's introduction in 1955, polio had been 97 percent eliminated in the United States. The era represented a high-water mark for American trust in institutions and authority figures.

But while most Americans in the years before the Covid pandemic reported feeling that the benefits of the measles vaccine outweighed any risks, and trusted scientists more than any other leadership group except the military, a small and loud community of vaccine skeptics had gained influence. Vaccination rates had declined in half of U.S. states during the previous decade, whether due to skepticism, lack of access, complacency about diseases that had largely disappeared precisely because of widespread vaccination, or some combination. Partly as a consequence, in 2019, the CDC recorded its highest number of measles cases since 1992, most of them among people who hadn't been vaccinated.

Though only a minority of Americans were hostile to the idea of vaccines in general, the story was different for the coming Covid vaccine in particular. Even as infections rose, Americans' willingness to take a vaccine declined. High-profile political figures, including then–vice presidential nominee Kamala Harris in October, declared they wouldn't trust a vaccine the president alone said was safe. The White House and the FDA engaged in a public tussle that same month over the agency's proposal for strict vaccine approval guidelines, which the president suggested were politically motivated, because they would delay approval until after the election. The Democratic governors of New York and California both announced that they'd appoint independent commissions in their states to review the vaccine's safety once it got FDA approval.

America's most important vaccine since polio was also the one Americans trusted least.

■   ■   ■

Sunday morning, November 15, Hamilton went out for a walk to try not to think about the meeting she had scheduled for 10:00 a.m. It was going to be a mighty Zoom gathering, with about 10 members of Hamilton's team, dozens of people working on vaccine-related issues from across the U.S. government, and an independent panel of experts—known as the Data and Safety Monitoring Board (DSMB)—all there to find out if Moderna's vaccine actually worked.

Everything she'd done for the past 10 months, all the 80-hour weeks and lost weekends and isolation—which went beyond social distancing, which was the isolation of knowing both that the world is relying on you and that almost nobody really understands what you're doing—all of that was on the line. She now saw her husband, whom she'd been with since she was 18, mostly in passing, walking to the coffee maker, as he was working from home, too. Long gone were the summer days where the two could take a 15-minute walk or eat lunch together. She ate meals at her desk and watched through the window when he left for his afternoon walks alone. *Oh, that's my husband. His beard looks good.* It was strange to miss someone who was in the same house with her at all times.

At least now she could have her own walk. Still, strolling through her neighborhood only forced her to focus on all the steps that had gotten her here. That Monday, November 9, Pfizer and BioNTech had announced the first efficacy breakthrough for a Covid vaccine. Hamilton had learned of the reveal early that morning, scrolling through email newsletters: In the Pfizer–BioNTech study, the overwhelming majority of people who ended up getting Covid had received a placebo shot, not the vaccine. Independent reviewers had determined the vaccine shot to be more than 90 percent effective in a preliminary analysis.

Her first feeling was a wave of relief. Pfizer's vaccine relied on the same kind of genetic technology that Moderna's did—indeed, that Moderna had based its whole corporate life on—and that prior to that very day had never been shown in clinical trials to effectively prevent disease in humans. And now, for the first time ever, an mRNA vaccine had been shown to work. To work far better than the 50 percent threshold necessary to get FDA approval, if the interim results held up. To work well enough to offer real hope of ending the pandemic.

Hamilton couldn't take much time to bask in the triumph for science or the hope for humanity. After all, this was a competitor's triumph. And while it provided early proof that Moderna's vaccine would work, too, Hamilton thought: *Okay, if they can do it, I know that we're going to be better. We have to be.*

. . . Right?

Six days later Hamilton came back from her morning walk, sat through a 45-minute presentation on safety data, and then commenced one of the longest hours of her life waiting for the monitoring board to meet separately to discuss the Moderna vaccine's fate. Hamilton buried herself in invoices. She couldn't control what they said. But she could control the drifts of administrative labor that kept swirling around her, by-products of running an enormous project she thought of as a small city. She texted a colleague to commiserate about the wait. He texted back a bit later to tell her: Get back on the call.

Hamilton found herself in a video chat room with colleagues, listening to a disembodied voice come through on a participant's speakerphone. The DSMB had invited Stephen Hoge, Moderna's president, and Anthony Fauci, the director of NIAID, which had partnered with Moderna from the beginning, to hear their first readout of the efficacy results. Hoge had put the DSMB meeting on speakerphone so that his colleagues could eavesdrop from another video chat room, and Hamilton logged on in time to hear a kind preamble from whichever review board member was speaking— this was a well-run study, you should be proud of the results, and so on. *Okay, okay, get to it*, she thought.

Finally, that voice started reading results. "Your efficacy is 94.5. Your case split is 90 and five." Of more than 30,000 people in the trials, 95 had gotten sick with Covid and displayed symptoms. Of those, fully 90 had been in the placebo group. Eleven severe cases had emerged in the study, none among the people who had taken the real vaccine.

Hamilton and her team hadn't just hit their goal—they'd walloped and smashed it. The Covid inoculation worked.

Hamilton was staring at her colleagues, all those faces in boxes on her laptop, everyone crying. One colleague kept turning off his video, presumably to collect himself; another clutched at a tissue. Hamilton wept, too. It was a rare scientific presentation that could bring tears, whether from relief, joy, or exhaustion. Hamilton could almost see the others get physically lighter, as the burden of uncertainty slid from each person's shoulders. They no longer had to carry their fear about how well it would work. It worked.

She heard Stephen thank the DSMB for their thorough review. And then she heard Anthony Fauci say: "All right. Now get to work."

But for the first time in weeks, Hamilton didn't have anything urgent she needed to do. She took the afternoon off. She ignored the piling emails from the few members of the company who, like her, had been briefed on the results—everyone else was going to have to wait for the formal announcement the company would make at 7:00 a.m. the next day. Those fortunate few dug into the data like eager puppies in snow, surfacing to toss new discoveries back and forth. *Did you see this table? Did you look at the case split post-dose one versus post-dose two? What about this evidence of preventing infection after the first dose?*

She was content to let them all nerd out without her. She cracked open a bottle of champagne and played a card game with her husband and their friend-family online. They did their traditional tarot reading.

Hamilton got a reversed moon. "Freeing yourself from limiting beliefs: the answers you seek are already inside you."

■   ■   ■

On December 7, 1941, 2,403 Americans died in the Japanese attack on Hawaii's Pearl Harbor naval base. The date was one President Franklin Delano Roosevelt said would live in infamy, and it pushed the United States into World War II.

On December 8, 2020, 2,661 Americans were reported dead from Covid. Yet across the ocean, at 6:31 a.m. local time at a hospital in Coventry, England, a nurse named May Parsons slipped a needle into the upper arm of Maggie Keenan, a retired jewelry shop assistant and a grandmother of four just a week shy of her 91st birthday. That date—V-Day in the United Kingdom—will live in honor as the beginning of the end of the global pandemic.

But the end would take a long time to arrive in the United States, and even the beginning of the end hadn't yet arrived when the first U.K.-approved vaccines got stuck into the first arms in England. The Pfizer vaccine Maggie received to applause from the assembled medical workers was still awaiting emergency authorization in the United States, having gotten it from U.K. regulators less than a week before.

Hamilton saw Maggie's picture in a news article but didn't have time to reflect on the gravity of the moment. The same was true when, on a Friday night, December 11, she was on the phone with a colleague trying to hash out the logistics of distributing the Moderna vaccine and got the notification that Pfizer's vaccine had been authorized for emergency use in the United States. It was world-shattering, eventually pandemic-ending news from which she moved on quickly, thinking that this at least made it unlikely the Moderna product would get rejected.

And finally, by the time doses of the Pfizer vaccine were packed in dry ice and loaded into trucks for distribution around the United States, and an ICU nurse in Queens named Sandra Lindsay became one of the first people in the country to get the shot on December 14, Hamilton was completely consumed with preparing for Moderna's own appeal for an emergency use authorization. On the same day that the vaccination drive kicked off in the United States—a milestone that General Gustave Perna, the chief operating officer of Operation Warp Speed, likened to the Normandy landings on D-Day, 1944—the Johns Hopkins ticker surpassed 300,000 in its count of American dead.

Her team was cramming into six weeks the six months' worth

of preparation that such a presentation would normally demand, spending full days of practice answering questions to ready themselves for the onslaught from the advisory committee that held the keys to authorization. Hamilton had declined the chance to be one of the people presenting the company's case, so instead was listening and jumping in with obnoxious notes: *you paused a little bit too long here,* or *you said we measured this in the throat but really we measured it in the nose and the lungs.* She knew her colleagues were perfectionists, and that the pressure weighed on them. She also knew that every word out of their mouths had to be precise.

■ ■ ■

Many different events then came together into a bundle of something that didn't quite add up to an ending. The FDA review panel, a group of independent experts who would advise regulators whether to approve the vaccine, held an eight-hour meeting on December 17, in pandemic style with floating heads on a screen. The gathering fizzled to an end after an interminable last-minute debate among the experts over whether to tweak the wording of the central question they'd convened to address: "Based on the totality of scientific evidence available, do the benefits of the Moderna COVID-19 Vaccine outweigh its risks for use in individuals 18 years of age and older?" No tweaks in the end.

Then the moderator, a jowly bald doctor in a candy-striped tie, put up a slide with the untweaked question for everyone to vote on—except that it was the slide about the Pfizer vaccine the panel had voted on a week before. Then a panelist pointed out the mistake. Then the correct slide went up. Then the panelists had two minutes to cast their votes. Then the votes rolled out. "Yes." "Yes." "Yes." "Yes." "Abstain." "Yes." "Yes." "Yes."

The final result was 20 Yesses and one abstention—from a panelist who objected to the wording of the question. They would resoundingly recommend emergency use authorization for Moderna's vaccine. The FDA took them up on the suggestion a day later, on December 18.

That night, after Moderna had its authorization in hand, Hamilton got on Zoom with members of the company's regulatory team, who had put together the reams of documentation necessary to make sense of Moderna's data and try to convince FDA to let people take their vaccine. This had meant assembling a data package for regulators and then fielding hundreds of questions about it, running new analyses or clarifying parts on request. As with the rest of the process, the team had been operating on a wildly compressed timeline.

Colleagues sipped white wine or champagne and Hamilton nursed a middle-grade bourbon, all of them barely believing that they'd survived to this point. The head of the team, Carla Vinals, recounted receiving the authorization letter from the FDA, rendered in the sterile language typical of a regulatory agency's dealings with a company. ("Having concluded that the criteria for issuance of this authorization under Section 564(c) of the Act are met, I am authorizing the emergency use of Moderna COVID-19 Vaccine for the prevention of COVID-19, as described in the Scope of Authorization section of this letter (Section II) and subject to the terms of this authorization . . .") Regulators eschewed warmth or chumminess in these kinds of communications; they were not supposed to be your friends, but independent arbiters. So it was a remarkable and powerful thing that Carla also got a nice note along with the authorization, lauding the achievements of the team, and the incredible value of their work to public health.

Regulators, it turned out, were people too.

On Monday morning Hamilton turned on the news. She was now used to seeing B-roll video of vaccine vials moving off production lines, with their yellow or gray or purple caps, but this time there was something different. Red caps. Moderna's color, which she'd never seen on stock footage before because the company had never produced vaccines at such a scale. Now she could see thousands of them rolling out, getting put into cartons with Moderna's name on them, to roll onto airplanes bound for rural communities neglected in earlier Pfizer vaccine shipments because of the Pfizer product's more-complicated storage requirements. Though the Pfizer and Moderna vaccines worked basically the same way with roughly the same efficacy—and in fact new data showed Pfizer's vaccine to be 95 percent effective in studies, almost exactly Moderna's rate—Pfizer's formula was then thought to require Antarctic-level ultra-cold storage of −94 degrees Fahrenheit, well beyond the capacity of a normal freezer, to keep the mRNA stable. Moderna's technology could keep the mRNA stable in a regular freezer at −4 degrees, which greatly simplified the process of shipping and storing. Hamilton knew that the results of her work would get to people so often neglected in public health, and that she and her team had actually done what they'd set out to do. They'd created a vaccine that was going to help millions of people, in the United States and in countries with far less sophisticated public-health infrastructure.

A few days later, on Christmas morning, she saw something even more moving. A colleague in Operation Warp Speed texted her a photo of a small group of maybe five or six people in a warehouse, standing in a circle around a case of the Moderna vaccine, blessing it.

■   ■   ■

To the extent Hamilton allowed herself to feel any sense of triumph, it was short-lived. The demands of U.S. regulators quickly gave way to the demands of European ones, who started launching their own volleys of hundreds of questions. Meanwhile, the U.S. rollout was proceeding more slowly than promised. The leadership of Operation Warp Speed had vowed 20 million inoculations in December, enough to hopefully start protecting most of the country's health-care workers and nursing home residents. But by January 1 federal data recorded that only about 12 million doses had been shipped and about 3 million actually administered, as states and hospitals navigated complicated logistics, conflicting guidance, and understaffing.

Scientists such as Hamilton had achieved miracles in getting a vaccine developed and tested so quickly, Operation Warp Speed had provided critical financial and logistical support to help them get there, and regulators had moved with incredible swiftness to ensure the product's safety. The whole process had been a triumph of private innovation and federal cooperation that, even with its snags and annoyances, showed how the U.S. government should act in an emergency. But now, nearly a year into America's pandemic, the best hope to stop it was getting ensnared in some of the very same dynamics that had assisted Covid's rampage through the country to begin with: The federal government was again foisting onto states responsibility without resources. Operation Warp Speed would mobilize the spectacular logistics of the U.S. military to get doses to states and then effectively walk away, leaving state health systems, many of them cash-strapped and overwhelmed, to get the shots into people's arms.

The results were predictable: long lines; crashing sign-up sites; some localities reporting too few doses and some too many. Hamilton watched all this with a sense of extreme frustration. Clinical sites in rural areas, places that had been on the front lines of the research and were bringing thousands of people through their doors during a global pandemic to help save others, now couldn't get access to vaccines to protect their staff and the subjects who had taken placebos. They had risked their own health in the service of testing a vaccine that they couldn't get, while some of the people Hamilton worked with in the government, who didn't even interact with the public, were getting shots themselves.

But then things began to shift. Moderna and Pfizer found ways to speed up manufacturing; the federal government struck deals with pharmacies around the country to help distribute vaccines, increased funding to states and urged them to expand access, and released doses held in reserve for second shots. President-elect Joe Biden was vowing to ramp up the rollout even further once he took office. Hamilton wanted to make sure, before taking the shot herself, that placebo recipients from the Moderna study all had access to the vaccine if they wanted it, and by January they could.

So on January 10, 2021, almost exactly a year from when she first saw the sequence of the new coronavirus and everything changed, Hamilton went with her husband to get the first dose of the shot she'd helped invent.

She knew, though, that she wasn't done, and in some ways the year that was beginning resembled the start of the year she'd left behind. Moderna needed to test its vaccine in adolescents now, and new variants of the virus demanded new research and new trials to make sure the vaccine could work against them too.

What she wanted now was the same thing she'd wanted since she first saw that string of letters that spelled out the viral genome a year ago: To go faster.

The Funeral Director

Last Responder

T HE VACCINE ROLLOUT did go faster, but so did the virus. America's first pandemic year of 2020 had ended in triumph with two vaccines authorized in December, and in devastation with a record 77,000 people perishing the same month. America's second pandemic year of 2021 had begun with hope and nearly 30 million vaccines administered by the end of January, and with anguish in the deadliest month of Covid yet for the country: More than 95,000 people who had survived through New Year's wouldn't live to see Valentine's Day.

It fell to funeral directors such as Jeff Jorgenson to take care of their bodies.

Jeff had witnessed the very start of Covid's American killing spree when some of the first victims showed up at the two West Coast funeral homes he helped operate, one in Washington where he lived, and one in California where he commuted a few times a month. Unexpectedly, considering his job, his most profound contact with the start of the U.S. pandemic involved not death but new life. His baby son was born on March 6 in Kirkland's Evergreen Hospital, which was even then becoming a Covid hot spot as it took patients from the nation's first nursing-home outbreak at the Life Care Center nearby. He and his mother-in-law were there to welcome little Robert's arrival into a strange world getting stranger. Within days, the hospital slammed shut its doors to visitors.

Now in January 2021, with the end of the pandemic supposedly in sight, Covid's killing had cruelly picked up speed. For the first time in his 15 years in the funeral industry, Jeff was turning families away. He had no place to put their dead.

Yet for the pandemic's first nine months or so, his business had been surprisingly slow. During that period Jeff had absorbed many jokes along the lines of "Wow, Covid must be great for you!" and his answer was always, "No, not really." Not just because Jeff, though his business was death, didn't actually root for it—but also because with so many people taking steps to avoid Covid, they were also avoiding other sicknesses that could kill them. Washington and California both had taken swift and severe measures to contain the virus, and early on at least, it showed. In revenue terms this was bad news for his funeral homes—and most other businesses—but good news for humanity. In Jeff's eyes people were genuinely doing the best they could not to get sick.

And there were some things that the pandemic hadn't changed at all. The needs of a family that had lost a father, mother, brother, sister, son, or daughter from Covid were the same as the needs of any family after death struck. Addressing those needs was part of what Jeff loved about the funeral business: When people were enduring some of life's worst pain, the bar was actually pretty low to make them happy. All you needed to do was make it not feel worse.

And sure there were different ways to do that, whether that involved making cremation or burial more affordable or offering advice on a motorcycle-themed service for someone's Harley-loving dad. But fundamentally all newly grieving families were alike in an important respect: They needed someone to help them put to rest a dead person they had loved.

What the pandemic did change was not this basic need but the ways in which Jeff and his colleagues could accommodate it. The first cases and deaths in Washington and California brought some of the first nationwide state shutdowns, and even though Jeff wasn't yet seeing many deaths from Covid, he also couldn't hold proper services for people who had died for other reasons. He knew that the right thing to do from a scientific perspective was to limit gatherings or forbid them altogether, but how was he supposed to tell that to someone whose mom had just died? How could he explain that the rules applied to the heartbroken, too?

The families he served mostly understood. But Jeff was losing some of his power to help them not feel worse.

Still, he managed. He got used to the restrictions. Neither the Seattle funeral home where he served on the front line of death care, nor the Los Angeles one he now helped run remotely due to travel restrictions, suffered the fate of overwhelmed funeral homes elsewhere as cascading death tolls shifted around the country through the spring and summer of 2020: New York, New Jersey, Michigan, Texas. Both California and Washington seemed to slow the spread of infection before the summer, but summer spikes in those states didn't strain his resources either. The deluge was still coming.

In winter, it hit.

It hit with special ferocity in Los Angeles, as if Covid somehow sensed the vaccine coming and was rushing to finish its fatal undertaking, before time ran out. A surge brought on in part by holiday travel and an innocent love for company generated hundreds of deaths per day in Los Angeles County alone by late January, more than quadruple the county's worst prior peak; 4,500 people had died there from New Year's Eve to January 22. The bodies were so numerous that officials lifted air-quality restrictions on cremations.

In Seattle, Jeff tried to manage the logistics of so much death in L.A. His California facility could store maybe 150 bodies, about 100 fewer people than the county was losing daily in late January. He tried to find more cooler space, but even some of the bigger facilities were full; he was calling as far away as Santa Barbara just to find room. The chaos was self-reinforcing: Doctors overwhelmed with trying to save people also faced a backlog of death certificates to sign; without a signed death certificate, a funeral home couldn't get a permit to bury or cremate; bodies remained in coolers for weeks at a time while families waited on paperwork.

Bereaved families were meanwhile calling Jeff constantly. Some burst into tears on the line just because someone had answered after they'd spent hours phoning funeral homes trying to find anybody who could help. Jeff usually couldn't help; he could show compassion but he couldn't conjure cooler space. Once or twice he cried at his desk himself. He was used to death, to processing death certificates and shielding himself from the thought that each was attached to a life lived and a person loved. He would have gone crazy otherwise. Every once in a while he'd share tears with a family whose story moved him. But he couldn't remember ever having cried over the sheer futility of his job, the pure and raw inability to do what he was there to do.

Sometimes, though, he and his colleagues did it. When a Salvadoran family called about a death at their home in January, Jeff's mortuary had room, and he started to chase down a death certificate. The man had lived with his mother and brother, and Jeff was relying on the brother to provide the personal and health information needed to get the documents in order for permission to cremate. But before Jeff could finish, the deceased man's brother was hospitalized with Covid, then intubated, and then died himself. Both brothers, then, wound up in the same cooler, their cremations delayed until Jeff's team was finally able to obtain the necessary permits. The timing worked out so that the brothers were cremated together on the same day.

This was a tiny point of solace for a suffering family. Comfort in the ashes. Peace for two brothers.

So Jeff spent every day dealing with the end of life and came home every night to life's beginning. Little Robert grew. He scooted, he crawled, he stood on his own, he babbled and laughed. And he grew.

It was proof that after the ashes, there would be more life.

Epilogue

L IFE, FOR ME, came back like an old friend. I'd lost touch with her for too long, but we resumed our old rhythms so easily I could almost feel like no time had passed. What I'd missed and appreciated about her—hugs and handshakes and casual chats with strangers, wide smiles unmasked—I quickly started taking for granted. And I soon rediscovered her forgotten flaws, the burdens of proximity to other people, the annoyances of social obligations I'd recently sworn I would cherish if I could just have them again.

The recovery happened to us one by one, or not at all. We lurched into a post-vaccine summer in 2021, by which time 150 million were vaccinated and 600,000 had died in the United States, a toll that would surpass 700,000 by year's end. We watched the virus ravage countries that lacked our vaccines, even as we, the American survivors, went on vacations or stayed hunkered down; we made up for lost time with friends or discovered we didn't want to; we went back to work or tried to avoid it or didn't have jobs to go back to or had never stopped going at all. Newspaper advice columns shifted attention, from coping with isolation to dealing with company. The mass layoffs of 2020 became the worker shortage of 2021; fears of another Great Depression became worries about inflation.

And still the virus wasn't fully vanquished, and still, just as in Camus's *The Plague*, the end of the story here can't be one of "final victory." His plague bacillus "never dies or disappears for good"; it lurks for years "in furniture and linen-chests . . . in bedrooms, cellars, trunks, and bookshelves," biding its time to "rouse up its rats again and send them forth to die in a happy city." Our coronavirus continues to spread, in America and around the world; it dwells in people's lungs and in the air around them, and in monkeys, cats, deer, and mink; it morphs into new variants and finds new victims; it courses through undervaccinated parts of the United States where people either refuse or can't get shots.

What meets it still is the stubborn spirit that drove the people in this book to help others. In place of victory is ongoing struggle, never finished, never enough. You can never save enough people, you can never make or distribute a vaccine fast enough or convince enough people to take it, you can never feed all of the hungry. But there are people who look those odds in the eye and try anyway.

They do this even when their elected leadership and public institutions fail them; they chase down the resources to save lives while politicians bicker and buck-pass and evade responsibility, and fellow citizens turn on each other. As much as this book is a story about individual heroism, it is also by implication an indictment of the institutions that left them unsupported or unprotected, and whose failures made so much of their courage necessary in the first place.

At the same time, *The Helpers* isn't a partisan morality tale. The virus further polarized a deeply politically divided country, but it also didn't care which side of the divide its victims fell on. Nor did the helpers described here: They include Trump supporters and socialists, and no one is worried about anyone else's party affiliation in the ICU or at the food pantry. Even at our most divided, our country is so much bigger and better than our politics.

Around the new year in 2021, when we'd all put our despised 2020 behind us but not yet our pandemic, I asked the helpers in this book what they'd learned in their separate fights with the virus and its effects. Everyone was ambivalent or modest in the lessons they drew. Hamilton Bennett reflected on how much the pandemic had taken from everyone, and on resilience in the face of loss. Chris Kiple, ever the CEO, had found new appreciation for a vital mission and teamwork; Huy Le wanted to find ways to live a more meaningful life. Michelle Gonzalez was happy to be alive and angry at institutions and leaders she thought had refused to care for the vulnerable or fix their obvious problems; Nikkia Rhodes stayed committed to gradual change in her community and to raising up the next generation of Black leaders. I never got to speak to Paul Cary, but I often think of what one of his colleagues told me about his attitude: That even facing the certainty of losing, you still show up to play. The helpers who are still with us told me about their hope for an eventually better future and the way love is heightened by the prospect of loss, the way gratitude intensifies when deprivation is all around.

I admit I wanted something bigger and more sense-making

about human nature, and Americans' nature in particular. Surely the ideas of gratitude and striving and teamwork couldn't be it. But as I kept thinking about it, I realized that really was it. We suffered on a grand scale and coped on a small one. Most of us tried and many of us failed. Some risked everything to save other people; we, the helped, owe our gratitude and in some cases our very lives to them.

In *The Plague*, Camus winds up modestly but stubbornly hopeful about human beings, a conclusion that strikes me as appropriate to the scale of human capabilities. His protagonist Dr. Rieux watches the fireworks of a city finally liberated from pestilence and reflects that, absent victory, his "could be only the record of what had to be done, and what assuredly would have to be done again in the never-ending fight against terror and its relentless onslaughts, despite their personal afflictions, by all who, while unable to be saints but refusing to bow down to pestilences, strive their utmost to be healers."

ACKNOWLEDGMENTS

THIS BOOK SIMPLY WOULD NOT exist if not for Bridget Matzie, who had the idea for it while out for a walk sometime in March 2020 and, for reasons I'm still not sure I get, thought I should do it. We'd never spoken before; I got her email while isolating and probably crying in my apartment, having just joined the growing ranks of Americans getting dumped in the pandemic. I did not get the proposal I expected in 2020, but because of Bridget I did write a book proposal, which was much better. Bridget, as Hall & Oates once said, you make my dreams come true.

Thanks to my fiendishly sharp editors Helen Thomaides, who was sharp and patient with the first draft, and John Glusman, who took a chance on an unknown writer. Shayna Elliot, Barbara Cohen, and Christopher Curioli provided indispensable help.

Thanks to Chris Cary, who was so generous in sharing his dad's story, and then his friendship and advice and humor, with me; and thank you to the rest of the Cary family, especially Sue and Sean. Thank you to Michelle Gonzalez, who showed me the Bronx; to Huy Le, who shares my love of Taylor Swift; to Chris Kiple, a fellow midwesterner who still owes me a beer; and to Nikkia Rhodes, whose cheerful wisdom is far beyond her 20-some-odd years and will stick with me. Thank you to Dr. Suzanne Pham of Weiss for her reflections on a painful time, and to Karyn Zielinski for facilitating those conversations and tracking down data. Thank you Scotty Hauser for introducing me, in his stories, to Charles. Thank you to Jeff Jorgenson for his surprisingly uplifting insights on the funeral industry. Thank you to Penny McGlachlin, who shared with me the story of her grandfather, A. W. "Smokey" Linn, and how he came to write the Fireman's Prayer.

Thanks to Hamilton Bennett, who gave generously of her Sundays to explain her historic work and put science into terms this layest of laypeople could understand. And to other members of the Moderna team who took the time, in the thick of the vaccine race, to tell me what they were up to: Stephane Bancel, Tal Zaks, and Stephen Hoge. But especially to Ray Jordan and Nancy McAdams, without whom none of this would have happened.

It's a great blessing to count some of my favorite writers among my best friends. This includes Julia Ioffe, who astonishes me with her capacity for generosity and humor and filthy rap lyrics. Olga Khazan talked me off numerous ledges, sent cookies at an especially hard time, and has in general made the toughest moments at work tolerable or at least funny. Adam Chandler put me up in Yonkers, shared Emily Saladino and Arby, and let me drive the Volvo around the

Bronx. And what can anyone even say about Jeff Stern, who has given me almost a decade's worth of laughter and guidance and Wednesday Night Beers, plus a whole month on the Jersey Shore, and who always knows just the right thing to say to scare off the doubt monster.

Thanks to Kate Stepleton, who has been my friend, role model, therapist, and co-conspirator since middle school, and whose text messages make me jealous of her writing. Thanks to Vance Serchuk, who's helped me think through the promise of America and encouraged me to recognize how much better we are than our terrible politics. Thanks to Jack Detsch for reading and helping me fix the first draft, for all the pep texts, and for enabling some of my worst habits.

Thanks to Amanda Givens for being a friend since my very first day on this planet, for remaining two days older than me, and for outgrowing a middle school phase involving a nu metal band I won't name here. Along with Amanda, thanks to Jason Givens (and Charlie, Louie, and Rose) and to Katie Flaschar, for the Patio Wine Nights (PWNs) that eased the isolation of 2020.

Thanks to the other friends who eased this process, especially Bo and Blake Simmons, Tom D'Arminio, Dan and Kaitlin Foster, Colin Gilboy, Valerie Martin, Mary Beth and Kevin Gilboy, Ariane Tabatabai, Merav Ceren, Karim Sadjadpour, Steven A. Cook, and David Singerman.

Thanks to the friends who are experts in various fields and who let me ask my dumb questions about science and medicine: Bharat

Reddy, Robin Kramer, Claire Mazumdar, Abby West (via the wonderful Andy Halterman), Emily Aaronson, and Avi Zenilman.

Thanks to the entire Kleinman family—my siblings from other mothers Emily and Stefan, Arielle and Andy, Madeleine and Taylor, Danny and Jenny; my de facto nephews Milo, Thomas, and Max; and my adopted parents Anne-Marie and Ron, who let me shelter in their house for months, and fed me, while I wrote the book proposal and whined about my feelings. Thank you Anne-Marie for all the virtual workout sessions with 202Strong and for the green smoothies and "Date Lab" readings on Saturdays. Ron, thanks for taking in the daughter you never wanted and for not kicking me out, but please don't worry: I'll be back.

And finally thank you infinity times to my family—Aunt Pat and Uncle Ken, who saw me through years in D.C. with the benefit of a few Manhattans; my brother and sister-in-law Jim and Jing, who sometimes laugh at my jokes at Zoom happy hours, but who always share my love of Mom's planning/organizational skills and Dad's gravy. Mom and Dad put me up while I wrote this and kept me fed and feeling loved. I told them Martha Gellhorn used to go back to St. Louis to write her books, but I doubt that her dad ever made such a good Rob Roy. I will always be grateful for walking around the block with Mom and seeing the penguins at the zoo, for "chef's night in" and Pepper O'Clock and *Better Call Saul*, for the kick-ass basement setup during quarantine and beyond, and for getting to call my own parents my favorite people. I mean, who *does* that?

NOTES

INTRODUCTION

xiv **forced to ration care:** Lucia Craxi, Marco Vergano, Julian Savulescu, and Dominic Wilkinson, "Rationing in a Pandemic: Lessons from Italy." *Asian Bioethics Review*. Vol. 12, No. 3 (September 2020), pp. 325–330. Published online June 16, 2020. Site: https://www.ncbi.nlm .nih.gov/pmc/articles/PMC7298692/.

xiv **15 confirmed instances in mid-February:** "CDC Confirms 15th Case of Coronavirus Disease." Centers for Disease Control and Prevention. February 13, 2020. Site: https://www.cdc .gov/media/releases/2020/s0213-15th-coronavirus-case.html.

xiv **1,000 in less than a month:** Will Feuer, "U.S. Coronavirus Cases Surpass 1,000, Up Nearly Ten-Fold in a Week." CNBC. March 10, 2020. Site: https://www.cnbc.com/2020/03/11/us -coronavirus-cases-surpass-1000-johns-hopkins-university-data-shows.html.

xiv **at least three months:** Lynsey Jeffery, "U.S. Surpasses 1 Million Coronavirus Cases." NPR. April 28, 2020. Site: https://www.npr.org/sections/coronavirus-live-updates/2020/04/28/846741935/u -s-surpasses-1-million-coronavirus-cases.

xiv **only 10 days:** VOA News, "U.S. Records 1 Million Covid-19 Cases in First 10 Days of November." Voice of America. November 10, 2020. Site: https://www.voanews.com/covid-19 -pandemic/us-records-1-million-covid-19-cases-first-10-days-november.

xiv **California shut down:** Gavin Newsom, "Executive Order N-33-20." Executive Department, State of California. March 19, 2020. Site: https://covid19.ca.gov/img/Executive-Order-N-33 -20.pdf.

xiv **the pandemic's global epicenter:** Donald G. McNeil, Jr., "The U.S. Now Leads the World in Confirmed Coronavirus Cases." *New York Times.* March 26, 2020. Site: https://www.nytimes .com/2020/03/26/health/usa-coronavirus-cases.html.

xiv **totally under control:** Matthew J. Belvedere, "Trump Says He Trusts China's Xi on Coronavirus and the U.S. Has It 'Totally Under Control.'" CNBC. January 22, 2020. Site: https:// www.cnbc.com/2020/01/22/trump-on-coronavirus-from-china-we-have-it-totally-under -control.html.

xiv **quarter of a million deaths:** Berkeley Lovelace, Jr., and Dan Mangan, "White House Predicts 100,000 to 240,000 Will Die in U.S. From Coronavirus." CNBC. March 31, 2020. Site: https://www.cnbc.com/2020/03/31/trump-says-the-coronavirus-surge-is-coming-its-going-to-be-a-very-very-painful-two-weeks.html.

xiv **more than 340,000:** Reuters Staff, "U.S. CDC Reports Record 3,764 Coronavirus Deaths in a Day." Reuters. December 31, 2020. Site: https://www.reuters.com/article/us-health-coronavirus-usa-cdc/u-s-cdc-reports-record-3764-coronavirus-deaths-in-a-day-idUSKBN2951RI.

xiv **pen-pal programs with nursing homes:** Cathy Free, "Residents at This Senior Center Asked for Pen Pals. They've Gotten Nearly 20,000 Letters." *Washington Post.* July 16, 2020. Site: https://www.washingtonpost.com/lifestyle/2020/07/16/pen-pal-letters-victorian-senior-care-covid/; and Cassie Hudson, "To Help Curb Loneliness, Cornell Students Create 'Quarantine Buddy.'" ABC News10. April 29, 2020. Site: https://www.news10.com/news/local-news/to-help-curb-loneliness-cornell-students-create-quarantine-buddy/.

xv **least productive in decades:** Neal Rothschild, "Productivity in Congress Tanked in 2020." *Axios.* December 14, 2020. Site: https://www.axios.com/congress-legislation-covid-19-2020-28a81b79-8cfc-4fc6-8fa6-e1758dd5f81f.html.

xv **more than $2 trillion:** Emily Cochrane and Sheryl Gay Stolberg, "$2 Trillion Coronavirus Stimulus Bill Is Signed into Law." *New York Times.* March 27, 2020. Site: https://www.nytimes.com/2020/03/27/us/politics/coronavirus-house-voting.html.

xv **overwhelmed blood banks:** Raymond Hernandez, "DONATIONS; Getting Too Much of a Good Thing." *New York Times.* November 12, 2001. Site: https://www.nytimes.com/2001/11/12/giving/donations-getting-too-much-of-a-good-thing.html.

xvi **enjoy our lives:** "President Holds Prime Time News Conference." Office of the Press Secretary. October 11, 2001. Site: https://georgewbush-whitehouse.archives.gov/news/releases/2001/10/20011011-7.html; and "At O'Hare, President Says 'Get on Board.'" Office of the Press Secretary. September 27, 2001. Site: https://georgewbush-whitehouse.archives.gov/news/releases/2001/09/20010927-1.html.

xvi **millions of people:** Paul Kiel, "The Great American Foreclosure Story: The Struggle for Justice and a Place to Call Home." *ProPublica.* April 10, 2012. Site: https://www.propublica.org/article/the-great-american-foreclosure-story-the-struggle-for-justice-and-a-place-t.

xvi **collective sense of purpose:** James M. Bickley, "War Bonds in the Second World War: A Model for a New War Bond?" Congressional Research Service. January 8, 2002. Site: https://fas.org/sgp/crs/misc/RS21046.pdf.

xvii **10 million net jobs lost:** Abigail Hess, "The U.S. Still Has 10 Million Fewer Jobs Now Than Before the Pandemic." CNBC. December 8, 2020. Site: https://www.cnbc.com/2020/12/08/the-us-has-10-million-fewer-jobs-now-than-before-the-pandemic.html.

xvii **record drug overdose deaths:** "Overdose Deaths Accelerating During Covid-19." Centers for Disease Control and Prevention. December 17, 2020. Site: https://www.cdc.gov/media/releases/2020/p1218-overdose-deaths-covid-19.html.

xvii **health officials went door-to-door:** Emma Graham-Harrison and Lily Kuo, "China's Coronavirus Lockdown Strategy: Brutal but Effective." *The Guardian.* March 19, 2020. Site: https://www.theguardian.com/world/2020/mar/19/chinas-coronavirus-lockdown-strategy-brutal-but-effective.

xvii **people had to carry forms:** "Attestations: The Three Permission Forms You Need in France to Leave Your Home." *The Local.* November 2, 2020. Site: https://www.thelocal.fr/20201102/attestations-the-three-permission-forms-you-need-to-leave-your-home-in-france.

xviii **most Americans reported:** Steve Crabtree, "Americans' Social Distancing Habits Have Tapered Since July." Gallup. October 19, 2020. Site: https://news.gallup.com/poll/322064/americans-social-distancing-habits-tapered-july.aspx.

xviii **"heroes of the highway":** Patrick McGee, "Outbreak Makes America's Truckers Heroes of the Highway." *Financial Times.* March 30, 2020. Site: https://www.ft.com/content/690f3fb3-2da1-4d65-9f6d-47be28ebdd3f.

xx **The president promulgated modest plans:** "15 Days to Slow the Spread." The White House. March 16, 2020. Site: https://www.whitehouse.gov/articles/15-days-slow-spread/.

xxi **"their certitude":** Albert Camus, *The Plague.* First Vintage International Edition. New York: Vintage Books, 1991, p. 133.

xxii **"There's no question of heroism":** Camus, *Plague,* p. 163.

xxii **laid the groundwork:** Annette McDermott, "Did World War II Launch the Civil Rights Movement?" History.com. January 31, 2021. Site: https://www.history.com/news/did-world-war-ii-launch-the-civil-rights-movement; and Annette McDermott, "How World War II Empowered Women." History.com. October 10, 2018. Site: https://www.history.com/news/how-world-war-ii-empowered-women.

PART ONE
THE PATIENT: SICK

4 **Facebook had asked its workers:** Reuters Staff, "Facebook, Google Ask San Francisco Staff to Work from Home as Coronavirus Spreads." Reuters. March 6, 2020. Site: https://www.reuters.com/article/us-healthcare-coronavirus-facebook/facebook-google-ask-san-francisco-staff-to-work-from-home-as-coronavirus-spreads-idUSKBN20T0LX.

5 **Both of those stricken:** John Woolfolk, "Santa Clara County Declares Its First Coronavirus Case Fully Recovered." *Mercury News.* February 20, 2020. Site: https://www.mercurynews.com/2020/02/20/santa-clara-county-declares-first-coronavirus-case-fully-recovered/.

5 **32 cases:** Bay City News, "Santa Clara County Reports 8 New Coronavirus Cases Saturday." NBC Bay Area. March 7, 2020. Site: https://www.nbcbayarea.com/news/local/south-bay/santa-clara-county-reports-8-new-coronavirus-cases-saturday/2249896/.

5 **first person to have died of Covid in the Bay Area:** Anna Bauman, "She Was the Last Person They Thought Could Have Coronavirus—and Among the First to Die in Bay Area." *San Francisco Chronicle.* March 26, 2020. Site: https://www.sfchronicle.com/bayarea/article/She-was-the-last-person-they-thought-could-have-15157910.php.

6 **quarantine on military bases:** Anita Chabria, Hannah Fry, and Jaclyn Cosgrove, "What We Know Now That Grand Princess Has Docked and Coronavirus Quarantines Have Begun." *Los Angeles Times.* March 11, 2020. Site: https://www.latimes.com/california/story/2020-03-09/what-we-know-about-grand-princess-docking-coronavirus-quarantine. See also: John Woolfolk, Julia Prodis Sulek, and Thy Vo, "Coronavirus: What Happens When Cruise Ship with Exposed Passengers Reaches San Francisco?" *Mercury News.* March 5, 2020. Site: https://www.mercurynews.com/2020/03/05/coronavirus-what-happens-when-cruise-ship-with-exposed-passengers-reaches-san-francisco/.

6 **first known Covid death:** David DeBolt, Fiona Kelliher, and Jason Green, "'She Held the Family Together:' San Jose Woman Is First Known U.S. Covid-19 Death." *Mercury News.* April 24, 2020. Site: https://www.mercurynews.com/2020/04/23/she-held-the-family-together-san-jose-woman-is-first-known-u-s-covid-19-death/.

6 **She hadn't traveled abroad:** Thomas Fuller, Mike Baker, Shawn Hubler, and Sheri Fink,

"A Coronavirus Death in Early February Was 'Probably the Tip of an Iceberg.'" *New York Times*. April 22, 2020. Site: https://www.nytimes.com/2020/04/22/us/santa-clara-county -coronavirus-death.html.

6 **conserve scarce tests:** Julie Small, "How the Nation's First COVID-19 Death Went Undetected in San Jose." KQED. May 4, 2020. Site: https://www.kqed.org/news/11816135/how-the -nations-first-covid-19-death-went-undetected-in-san-jose.

7 **survivors faced other dangers:** Chris McGreal, "Vietnamese Boat People: Living to Tell the Tale." *The Guardian*. March 19, 2020. Site: https://www.theguardian.com/global/2016/mar/20/ vietnamese-boat-people-survivors-families. See also: Thomas Van Nguyen, "The Price of Freedom." United States Army. June 4, 2015. Site: https://www.army.mil/article/149841/the_ price_of_freedom.

9 **a human hair:** Benedette Cufari, "The Size of SARS-CoV-2 Compared to Other Things." *News Medical*. July 16, 2020. Site: https://www.news-medical.net/health/The-Size-of-SARS -CoV-2-Compared-to-Other-Things.aspx.

11 **three-fourths of Americans:** "Coronavirus: Three Out of Four Americans Under Some Form of Lockdown." BBC News. March 31, 2020. Site: https://www.bbc.com/news/world-us -canada-52103066.

11 **at least 25 million people:** Tim Arango and Jill Cowan, "Gov. Newsom of California Orders Californians to Stay Home." *New York Times*. March 19, 2020. Site: https://www.nytimes .com/2020/03/19/us/California-stay-at-home-order-virus.html.

11 **"There is a social contract":** "California Governor Newsom Coronavirus News Conference." C-SPAN. March 19, 2020. Site: https://www.c-span.org/video/?470539-1/california -governor-newsom-coronavirus-news-conference.

13 **making it difficult to breathe:** "What Coronavirus Symptoms Look Like, Day By Day" [Video]. Science Insider. March 18, 2020. Site: https://www.youtube.com/watch?v=OOJqHPfG7pA.

THE VACCINE DEVELOPER: THE GAMBLE

16 **it wasn't unusual for Hamilton:** Hamilton Bennett, telephone interview by the author, November 29, 2020.

16 **infected nearly 60 people:** Fanfan Wang, Natasha Kan, and Rachel Yeo, "Health Officials Work to Solve China's Mystery Virus Outbreak." *Wall Street Journal*. January 6, 2020. Site: https://www.wsj.com/articles/health-officials-work-to-solve-chinas-mystery-virus-outbreak -11578308757.

16 **a city of 11 million:** Huizhong Wu and Sophie Yu, "China to Step Up Countermeasures as Virus Outbreak Grows." Reuters. January 18, 2020. Site: https://www.reuters.com/article/ us-china-health-pneumonia/china-to-step-up-countermeasures-as-virus-outbreak-grows -idUSKBN1ZI028.

16 **Reports recited statistics:** Donald G. McNeil, Jr. "Wuhan Coronavirus Looks Increasingly Like a Pandemic, Experts Say." *New York Times*. February 2, 2020. Site: https://www.nytimes .com/2020/02/02/health/coronavirus-pandemic-china.html.

17 **"It's impossible":** Xu Jianguo as quoted in Gerry Shih and Lena H. Sun, "Specter of Possible New Virus Emerging from Central China Raises Alarms Across Asia." *Washington Post*. January 8, 2020. Site: https://www.washingtonpost.com/world/asia_pacific/specter-of-possible -new-virus-emerging-from-central-china-raises-alarms-across-asia/2020/01/08/3d33046c -312f-11ea-971b-43bec3ff9860_story.html.

18 **"human cells into drug factories":** Damian Garde, "Ego, Ambition, and Turmoil: Inside

One of Biotech's Most Secretive Startups." *STAT.* September 13, 2016. Site: https://www
.statnews.com/2016/09/13/moderna-therapeutics-biotech-mrna/.

18 **Moderna executives evangelized:** Meg Tirrell, "The Biotech Targeting Personalized Medicine." CNBC. May 12, 2015. Site: https://www.cnbc.com/2015/05/12/moderna-therapeutics
-is-trying-to-cure-disease-with-mrna-drugs.html.

18 **could hurt the patient:** Damian Garde and Jonathan Salzman, "The Story of mRNA: How a
Once-Dismissed Idea Became a Leading Technology in the Covid Vaccine Race." *STAT, Boston Globe.* November 10, 2020. Site: https://www.statnews.com/2020/11/10/the-story-of-mrna
-how-a-once-dismissed-idea-became-a-leading-technology-in-the-covid-vaccine-race/.

18 **had largely given up:** Garde, "Ego, Ambition, and Turmoil."

19 **in just 60 days:** Robert Langreth and Naomi Kresge, "Moderna Wants to Transform the
Body into a Vaccine-Making Machine." *Bloomberg Businessweek.* August 11, 2020. Site: https://
www.bloomberg.com/features/2020-moderna-biontech-covid-shot/?srnd=businessweek-v2.

19 **more than two decades:** Claudi Kalb, "Dr. Paul Offit: Debunking the Vaccine-Autism Link."
Newsweek. October 24, 2020. Site: https://www.newsweek.com/dr-paul-offit-debunking
-vaccine-autism-link-91933.

19 **Most vaccines failed in development:** Nancy Schimelpfenig, "Many Early Vaccine Trials Show Promise. Most Still Fail. Here's Why." *Healthline.* July 30, 2020. Site: https://www
.healthline.com/health-news/many-early-vaccine-trials-show-promise-most-still-fail-heres
-why.

23 **confident about getting a vaccine:** Katie Thomas, "The Race for a Zika Vaccine." *New York
Times.* November 19, 2020. Site: https://www.nytimes.com/2016/11/20/business/testing-the
-limits-of-biotech-in-the-race-for-a-zika-vaccine.html?module=inline.

23 **a mere eight months:** Helen Branswell, "A Zika Vaccine Is Being Developed at Warp Speed,
but Will There Be a Market for It?" *STAT,* December 6, 2016. Site: https://www.statnews
.com/2016/12/05/zika-vaccine-development-market/.

25 **a new kind of coronavirus:** "WHO Statement Regarding Cluster of Pneumonia Cases in
Wuhan, China." World Health Organization. January 9, 2020. Site: https://www.who.int/
china/news/detail/09-01-2020-who-statement-regarding-cluster-of-pneumonia-cases-in
-wuhan-china.

25 **around 20 months:** Knvul Sheikh and Katie Thomas, "Researchers Are Racing to Make a
Coronavirus Vaccine. Will It Help?" *New York Times.* January 28, 2020. Site: https://www
.nytimes.com/2020/01/28/health/coronavirus-vaccine.html.

25 **eight years after MERS:** "NIH Clinical Trial of Investigational Vaccine for COVID-19
Begins." NIH. March 16, 2020. Site: https://www.nih.gov/news-events/news-releases/nih
-clinical-trial-investigational-vaccine-covid-19-begins.

25 **One researcher speculated:** Gerry Shih and Lena H. Sun, "China Identifies New Strain of
Coronavirus as Source of Pneumonia Outbreak." *Washington Post.* January 10, 2020. Site: https://
www.washingtonpost.com/world/asia_pacific/china-identifies-new-strain-of-coronavirus-as
-source-of-pneumonia-outbreak/2020/01/09/f2625650-329f-11ea-971b-43bec3ff9860_story
.html.

26 **30,000-odd letters long:** Fan Wu, Su Zhao, Bin Yu, Yan-Mei Chen, Wen Wang, Zhi-
Gang Song, Yi Hu, Zhao-Wu Tao, Jun-Hua Tian, Yuan-Yuan Pei, Ming-Li Yuan, Yu-Ling
Zhang, Fa-Hui Dai, Yi Liu, Qi-Min Wang, Jiao-Jiao Zheng, Lin Xu, Edward C. Holmes,
and Yong-Zhen Zhang, "Severe Acute Respiratory Syndrome Coronavirus 2 Isolate Wuhan-
Hu-1, Complete Genome." GenBank via NCBI. Site: https://www.ncbi.nlm.nih.gov/nuccore/
MN908947.

27 **sounded crazy to her:** Catherine Elton, "The Untold Story of Moderna's Race for a Covid-19 Vaccine." *Boston Magazine.* June 4, 2020. Site: https://www.bostonmagazine.com/health/2020/06/04/moderna-coronavirus-vaccine/.

28 **he launched a Web dashboard:** Kyle Swenson, "Millions Track the Pandemic on Johns Hopkins's Dashboard. Those Who Built It Say Some Miss the Real Story." *Washington Post.* June 29, 2020. Site: https://www.washingtonpost.com/local/johns-hopkins-tracker/2020/06/29/daea7eea-a03f-11ea-9590-1858a893bd59_story.html.

THE CEO: RAMPING UP

32 **He began to show symptoms:** KIRO 7 News Staff and Linzi Sheldon, "First Case of Covid-19 Confirmed in Snohomish County." KIRO7. January 21, 2020. Site: https://www.kiro7.com/news/local/report-announcement-expected-first-case-wuhan-coronavirus-washington/55H JS7WWFRD5ZB4INKJSILDIFI/.

32 **Trump shut down most travel:** Donald J. Trump, "Proclamation on Suspension of Entry as Immigrants and Nonimmigrants of Persons Who Pose a Risk of Transmitting the 2019 Novel Coronavirus." The White House. January 31, 2020. Site: https://trumpwhitehouse.archives .gov/presidential-actions/proclamation-suspension-entry-immigrants-nonimmigrants -persons-pose-risk-transmitting-2019-novel-coronavirus/.

32 **two-week federal quarantine:** Kathy Gilsinan, "Friendships in the Age of Quarantine." *The Atlantic.* March 15, 2020. Site: https://www.theatlantic.com/politics/archive/2020/03/social -distancing-coronavirus-quarantine-friendship/607942/.

32 **first known U.S. Covid death:** Nicole Acevedo and Minyvonne Burke, "Washington State Man Becomes First U.S. Death from Coronavirus." NBC News. February 29, 2020. Site: https://www.nbcnews.com/news/us-news/1st-coronavirus-death-u-s-officials-say-n1145931.

33 **142 COVID-19 cases:** Asia Fields and Mary Hudetz, "Coronavirus Spread at the Life Care Center for Weeks, While Response Stalled." *Seattle Times.* March 18, 2020. Site: https://www .seattletimes.com/seattle-news/times-watchdog/coronavirus-spread-in-a-kirkland-nursing -home-for-weeks-while-response-stalled/.

33 **a quarter of Covid fatalities:** Fields and Hudetz, "Coronavirus Spread at the Life Care Center for Weeks."

33 **The disease ultimately killed 39:** Heidi Pino, "Life Care Center of Kirkland Honors Residents Lost to Covid-19." Life Care Center of Kirkland. September 3, 2020. Site: https://lcca .com/locations/wa/kirkland/blog/COVID-19-memorial-service-kirkland.

33 **poor infection control:** Olga Khazan, "The U.S. Is Repeating Its Deadliest Pandemic Mistake." *The Atlantic.* July 6, 2020. Site: https://www.theatlantic.com/health/archive/2020/07/us -repeating-deadliest-pandemic-mistake-nursing-home-deaths/613855/.

34 **ordering ventilators by the thousands:** John Miller, "Germany, Italy Rush to Buy Life-Saving Ventilators as Manufacturers Warn of Shortages." Reuters. March 13, 2020. Site: https://www.reuters.com/article/us-health-coronavirus-draegerwerk-ventil/germany-italy -rush-to-buy-life-saving-ventilators-as-manufacturers-warn-of-shortages-idUSKBN210362.

34 **Italy had started rationing ventilators:** Lisa Rosenbaum, MD, "Facing Covid-19 in Italy— Ethics, Logistics, and Therapeutics on the Epidemic's Front Line." *New England Journal of Medicine.* Vol. 382 (March 18, 2020), pp. 1873–1875. Site: https://www.nejm.org/doi/full/10 .1056/nejmp2005492; and Mattia Ferraresi, "A Coronavirus Cautionary Tale from Italy: Don't Do What We Did." *Boston Globe.* March 13, 2020. Site: https://www.bostonglobe .com/2020/03/13/opinion/coronavirus-cautionary-tale-italy-dont-do-what-we-did/.

35 **national emergency:** Donald J. Trump, "Proclamation on Declaring a National Emergency Concerning the Novel Coronavirus Disease (Covid-19) Outbreak." The White House. March 13, 2020. Site: https://trumpwhitehouse.archives.gov/presidential-actions/proclamation -declaring-national-emergency-concerning-novel-coronavirus-disease-covid-19-outbreak/.

35 **"When patients' breathing deteriorates":** Robert D. Truog, MD, Christine Mitchell, RN, and George Q. Daly, MD, PhD, "The Toughest Triage—Allocating Ventilators in a Pandemic." *New England Journal of Medicine.* Vol. 382 (March 23, 2020), pp. 1973–1975. Site: https://www.nejm.org/doi/full/10.1056/nejmp2005689.

36 **47 deaths:** Jessie Yeung, Joshua Berlinger, Adam Renton, Meg Wagner, Mike Hayes, and Veronica Rocha, "March 13 Coronavirus News." CNN.com. March 13, 2020. Site: https:// www.cnn.com/world/live-news/coronavirus-outbreak-03-13-20-intl-hnk/index.html.

36 **"There will likely be":** "CDC Confirms 15th Case of Coronavirus Disease (Covid-19)." Centers for Disease Control and Prevention. February 13, 2020. Site: https://www.cdc.gov/media/ releases/2020/s0213-15th-coronavirus-case.html.

38 **donating his ventilator:** "Coronavirus: Hawking's Family Donate Ventilator to Hospital." BBC News. April 22, 2020. Site: https://www.bbc.com/news/uk-england-cambridgeshire -52380603#:~:text=Stephen%20Hawking's%20personal%20ventilator%20has,Royal%20 Papworth%20Hospital%20in%20Cambridge.

39 **60,000 full-featured ventilators:** Neil A. Halpern, MD, and Kay See Tan, PhD, "United States Resource Availability for Covid-19." Society of Critical Care Medicine. March 13, 2020, revised May 12, 2020. Site: https://www.sccm.org/getattachment/Blog/March-2020/ United-States-Resource-Availability-for-COVID-19/United-States-Resource-Availability -for-COVID-19.pdf?lang=en-US.

40 **an oft-cited guess:** Halpern and Tan, "United States Resource Availability for Covid-19."

40 **could kill 2.2 million:** Neil M. Ferguson, Daniel Laydon, Gemma Nedjati-Gilani, Natsuko Imai, Kylie Ainslie, Marc Baguelin, Sangeeta Bhatia, Adhiratha Boonyasiri, Zulma Cucunubá, Gina Cuomo-Dannenburg, Amy Dighe, Ilaria Dorigatti, Han Fu, Katy Gaythorpe, Will Green, Arran Hamlet, Wes Hinsley, Lucy C. Okell, Sabine van Elsland, Hayley Thompson, Robert Verity, Erik Volz, Haowei Wang, Yuanrong Wang, Patrick G.T. Walker, Caroline Walters, Peter Winskill, Charles Whittaker, Christl A. Donnelly, Steven Riley, and Azra C. Ghani, "Report 9: Impact of Non-pharmaceutical Interventions (NPIs) to Reduce Covid-19 Mortality and Healthcare Demand." Imperial College Covid Response Team. March 16, 2020. Site: https://www.imperial.ac.uk/media/imperial-college/medicine/sph/ide/gida -fellowships/Imperial-College-COVID19-NPI-modelling-16-03-2020.pdf.

40 **80,000 American deaths:** Christopher J.L. Murray, "Forecasting Covid-19 Impact on Hospital Bed-Days, Ventilator Days and Deaths By U.S. State in the Next 4 Months." *MedRxiv.* March 26, 2020. Site: http://www.healthdata.org/research-article/forecasting-covid-19 -impact-hospital-bed-days-icu-days-ventilator-days-and-deaths.

40 **tens of thousands:** Murray, "Forecasting Covid-19 Impact."

40 **The nationwide shortfall:** Cynthia McFadden, Kit Ramgopal, Lisa Cavazuti, Christine Romo, and Brenda Breslauer, "A Small Seattle Firm Is Working Around the Clock to Make Lifesaving Ventilators for Coronavirus Patients." NBC News. March 18, 2020. Site: https:// www.nbcnews.com/health/health-care/small-seattle-firm-working-around-clock-make-life -saving-ventilators-n1162951.

40 **40,000 to 50,000 units:** William Baldwin, "Ventilator Maker: We Can Ramp Up Production Five-Fold." *Forbes.* March 14, 2020. Site: https://www.forbes.com/sites/baldwin/2020/03/14/ ventilator-maker-we-can-ramp-up-production-five-fold/#5347b6df5e9a.

42   **Ventec could ramp up production:** Baldwin, "Ventilator Maker."
45   **custom built:** Dave Good, telephone interview by the author, November 19, 2020.

THE PARAMEDIC: ROAD TRIP

46   **snowstorm bearing down:** "Denver Weather: Cold Front Arrives This Evening, Rain and
     Snow Friday." CBS 4 Denver. March 26, 2020. Site: https://denver.cbslocal.com/2020/03/26/
     denver-weather-cold-front-arrives-rain-snow-colorado/.
47   **called the scene "apocalyptic":** Michael Rothfeld, Somini Sengupta, Joseph Goldstein, and
     Brian M. Rosenthal, "13 Deaths in a Day: An 'Apocalyptic' Coronavirus Surge at an N.Y.C.
     Hospital." *New York Times.* March 25, 2020. Site: https://www.nytimes.com/2020/03/25/
     nyregion/nyc-coronavirus-hospitals.html.
47   **joining 20 other states:** "When Stay-at-Home Orders Due to Coronavirus Went Into Ef-
     fect." Kaiser Family Foundation. April 9, 2020. Site: https://www.kff.org/other/slide/when
     -state-stay-at-home-orders-due-to-coronavirus-went-into-effect/.
47   **pleaded with residents:** Sam Tabachnik and Alex Burness, "Gov. Jared Polis Orders Colo-
     rado to Stay Home in Bid to Slow the Coronavirus Outbreak." *Denver Post.* March 25, 2020.
     Site: https://www.denverpost.com/2020/03/25/colorado-stay-at-home-coronavirus-polis/.
48   **Denver firefighter who had died:** U.S. Fire Administration, "Richard Patrick Mon-
     toya, Lieutenant." Date of death May 21, 2006. Site: https://apps.usfa.fema.gov/firefighter
     -fatalities/fatalityData/detail?fatalityId=3285.
50   **firehouse tradition with murky origins:** Sara Rimer, "The Fireman's Mustache: Badge of
     the Brotherhood." *New York Times.* June 21, 1986. Site: https://www.nytimes.com/1986/06/21/
     nyregion/the-fireman-s-mustache-badge-of-the-brotherhood.html#:~:text=The%20
     mustache%2C%20according%20to%20regulations,portion%20of%20the%20upper%20lip
     .&text=Firefighter%20Appiarius%2C%20who%20is%20assigned,traditionally%20came%20
     from%20the%20military.
51   **most advanced care available:** EMS1 Staff, "Paramedic vs. EMT: Which Path is Right for
     You?" *EMS1.* October 14, 2011. Site: https://www.ems1.com/ems-products/books/articles/
     paramedic-vs-emt-which-path-is-right-for-you-nSqJ5Z1ngroThrDy/.
51   **on a basement floor:** Celia Sporer, telephone interview by the author, July 20, 2020.
53   **aura of calm and purpose:** Danielle Wardrop, telephone interview by the author, August 4,
     2020.
55   **sometimes he would get sick:** Wardrop, telephone interview.
57   **United States had overtaken China:** Rebecca Liebson, "100 Coronavirus Deaths in One
     Day." *New York Times.* March 29, 2020. Site: https://www.nytimes.com/2020/03/27/nyregion/
     coronavirus-nyc.html.
57   **200 had already tested positive:** Ali Watkins, "N.Y.C.'s 911 System is Overwhelmed. 'I'm
     Terrified, A Paramedic Says." *New York Times.* March 28, 2020. Site: https://www.nytimes
     .com/2020/03/28/nyregion/nyc-coronavirus-ems.html.
57   **911 system took 5,700 calls:** Rachel Engel, "FDNY Hit Hard by COVID-19: EMS Chief
     Bonsignore Says Historic Call Volume Likely to Increase." *EMS1.* March 30, 2020. Site:
     https://www.ems1.com/fdny-ems/articles/fdny-hit-hard-by-covid-19-ems-chief-bonsignore
     -says-historic-call-volume-likely-to-increase-GhK6MKjwEvBAAQSf/.
57   **smashing its own records:** Watkins, "N.Y.C.'s 911 System Is Overwhelmed."

THE NURSE: THE WORST SHIFT

60 **"You pick the 26,000 people":** Shannon Young and Marie J. French, "Andrew Cuomo to Trump Administration: 'You Pick the 26K People Who Are Going to Die." *Politico.* March 24, 2020. Site: https://www.politico.com/states/new-york/albany/story/2020/03/24/cuomo-to-trump-administration-you-pick-the-26k-people-who-are-going-to-die-1268833.

61 **"TREATED LIKE TRASH":** Carl Capanile and Ebony Bowden, "Nurses at NYC Hospital Receive Gowns After Post Trash Bag Expose." *New York Post.* April 2, 2020. Site: https://nypost.com/2020/04/02/nurses-at-nyc-hospital-receive-gowns-after-post-trash-bag-expose/.

61 **staff started a GoFundMe drive:** "PPE for NYC's Montefiore Emergency Room Providers." GoFundMe. March 25, 2020. Site: https://www.gofundme.com/f/ppe-for-montefiore-emergency-room-providers.

61 **glue-gun face-shields together:** Eva Radke, "Meet Your Maker: Cat Navarro." ArtCube Army Blog. May 15, 2020. Site: https://www.artcubearmy.com/post/meet-your-maker-cat-navarro.

61 **"the patron saint of PPE":** Jada Yuan, "New York's Patron Saint of PPE Went $600,000 into Debt to Outfit Workers—and Hospitals Keep Turning Her Down." *Washington Post.* May 6, 2020. Site: https://www.washingtonpost.com/national/new-york-hospitals-ppe-rhonda-roland-shearer/2020/05/05/d8e4bc16-8bb6-11ea-8ac1-bfb250876b7a_story.html.

61 **"not a shipping clerk":** Quint Forgey, "'We're Not a Shipping Clerk': Trump Tells Governors to Step Up Efforts to Get Medical Supplies." *Politico,* March 19, 2020. Site: https://www.politico.com/news/2020/03/19/trump-governors-coronavirus-medical-supplies-137658.

61 **government had ignored early warnings:** Aaron C. Davis, "In the Early Days of the Pandemic, the U.S. Government Turned Down an Offer to Manufacture Millions of N95 Masks in America." *Washington Post,* May 9, 2020. Site: https://www.washingtonpost.com/investigations/in-the-early-days-of-the-pandemic-the-us-government-turned-down-an-offer-to-manufacture-millions-of-n95-masks-in-america/2020/05/09/f76a821e-908a-11ea-a9c0-73b93422d691_story.html.

61 **claiming domestic production for itself:** Zhuang Pinghui and Zhou Xin, "Coronavirus: China Shifts Responsibility Over Medical Supplies Amid Mask Shortage, Rising Death Toll." *South China Morning Post.* February 3, 2020. Site: https://www.scmp.com/economy/china-economy/article/3048744/coronavirus-mask-shortage-prompts-beijing-tweak-authority.

66 **two to nearly 700:** "First-of-Its-Kind Report Details How New York Children's Hospital Transformed to Provide Care to Adult Covid-19 Patients." Montefiore News Releases. May 20, 2020. Site: https://www.montefiore.org/body.cfm?id=1738&action=detail&ref=1737.

69 **highest confirmed rates of infection:** David Gonzalez, "'The City Fumbled It': How Four Families Took on the Virus." *New York Times.* June 24, 2020. Site: https://www.nytimes.com/2020/06/24/nyregion/coronavirus-public-housing-new-york.html.

69 **almost three times as likely:** Ese Olumhense and Ann Choi, "Bronx Residents Twice as Likely to Die from Covid in NYC." *The City.* April 3, 2020. Site: https://www.thecity.nyc/health/2020/4/3/21210372/bronx-residents-twice-as-likely-to-die-from-covid-19-in-nyc.

70 **was nicknamed "Asthma Alley":** Hazar Kilani, "'Asthma Alley': Why Minorities Bear the Burden of Pollution Inequity Caused by White People." *The Guardian.* Site: https://www.theguardian.com/us-news/2019/apr/04/new-york-south-bronx-minorities-pollution-inequity.

70 **the average life expectancy:** "Mott Haven and Melrose: Community Health Profiles 2018." Bronx Community District 1. Site: https://www1.nyc.gov/assets/doh/downloads/pdf/data/2018chp-bx1

.pdf; and "Upper East Side: Community Health Profiles 2018." Manhattan Community District 8. Site: https://www1.nyc.gov/assets/doh/downloads/pdf/data/2018chp-mn8.pdf.

70 **62nd, dead last:** "How New York Counties Rank on Health." *Newsday.* Site: https://projects .newsday.com/databases/long-island/new-york-counties-health-rank/.

70 **60 percent of Bronx residents:** "Bronx County, NY." Data USA. Site: https://datausa.io/ profile/geo/bronx-county-ny.

70 **the borough's own underlying conditions:** "Health Equity Considerations and Racial and Ethnic Minority Groups." Centers for Disease Control and Prevention. July 24, 2020. Site: https://www.cdc.gov/coronavirus/2019-ncov/community/health-equity/race-ethnicity .html?CDC_AA_refVal=https%3A%2F%2Fwww.cdc.gov%2Fcoronavirus%2F2019 -ncov%2Fneed-extra-precautions%2Fracial-ethnic-minorities.html.

70 **44-story public housing project:** Kimiko de Freytas-Tamura, Winnie Hu, and Lindsey Rogers Cook, "'It's the Death Towers': How the Bronx Became New York's Virus Hot Spot." *New York Times.* May 26, 2020. Site: https://www.nytimes.com/2020/05/26/nyregion/bronx -coronavirus-outbreak.html.

70 **a mom, a grandma, and six kids:** Kirstyn Brendlen, "Nurses Say No Masks, Gloves Only the Beginning." *Riverdale Press.* April 19, 2020. Site: https://riverdalepress.com/stories/nurses-say -no-masks-gloves-only-the-beginning,71656.

70 **commutes into and out of one Bronx neighborhood:** Winnie Hu and Nate Schweber, "When Rich New Yorkers Fled, These Workers Kept the City Running." *New York Times.* June 16, 2020. Site: https://www.nytimes.com/2020/06/16/nyregion/mount-hope-bronx -coronavirus-essential-workers.html.

73 **"home for chronic invalids":** "The Home for Chronic Invalids." *New York Times.* October 27, 1884. Site: https://timesmachine.nytimes.com/timesmachine/1884/10/27/106165167 .pdf?pdf_redirect=true&ip=0.

73 **blanket over his head:** Leonard Greene, "Overcrowding at Montefiore Is a Bitter Pill to Swallow for Nurses and Patients." *New York Daily News.* October 15, 2018. Site: https://www .nydailynews.com/new-york/ny-metro-nurses-hospital-hallways-20181015-story.html.

THE CHEF: SHUTDOWN

75 **aspiring nurse named Breonna Taylor:** Tessa Duval, "FACT CHECK 2.0: Debunking 9 Widely Shared Rumors in the Breonna Taylor Shooting." Louisville *Courier-Journal.* June 16, 2020. Site: https://www.courier-journal.com/story/news/crime/2020/06/16/breonna-taylor -fact-check-7-rumors-wrong/5326938002/.

76 **daily flights to China:** Grace Schneider, "UPS Says Coronavirus Is Already Cutting Demand and Disrupting Supply Chains." Louisville *Courier-Journal.* February 28, 2020. Site: https://www.courier-journal.com/story/money/companies/2020/02/28/ups-coronavirus -cuts-demand-customers-taking-hit-supply-chains/4905364002/.

76 **already in February:** Alfred Miller and Grace Schneider, "Coronavirus Fears Could Upend City's Derby Plans; Louisville Officials Prepare as Virus Spreads Across the Globe." Louisville *Courier-Journal.* February 24, 2020. Site: https://www.courier-journal.com/story/ money/companies/2020/02/24/coronavirus-fears-could-upend-louisvilles-kentucky-derby -plans/4860352002/.

76 **grocery chains were imposing caps:** Karla Ward, "Kroger Moves to Limit Hoarding of Sanitizers, Cold and Flu Meds Amid Coronavirus Worry." *Lexington Herald-Leader.* March 4, 2020. Site: https://www.kentucky.com/news/local/article240861291.html.

76 **"Kentuckians remain at low risk"**: "Gov. Beshear, Health Officials Confirm State's First Covid-19 Case." Office of the Governor. March 6, 2020. Site: https://kentucky.gov/Pages/Activity-stream.aspx?n=GovernorBeshear&prId=77.

77 **80 percent of Iroquois students:** "Iroquois Neighborhood Profile." Kentucky State Data Center and Metro United Way. July 2017. Site: http://ksdc.louisville.edu/wp-content/uploads/2018/06/Iroquois.pdf.

79 **one of two:** John P. Wise, "Friday the 13th Ends with Second Deadly LMPD-Involved Shooting in Less Than 24 Hours." WAVE3 News. March 13, 2020. Site: https://www.wave3.com/2020/03/14/friday-th-ends-with-second-deadly-lmpd-involved-shooting-less-than-hours/.

79 **murder rate was rising:** Sarah Ladd and Billy Kobin, "'It's Like a Repeated Cycle': Louisville's Murder Toll Climbed 14% in 2019." Louisville *Courier-Journal*. January 3, 2020. Site: https://www.courier-journal.com/story/news/crime/2020/01/03/how-much-louisville-homicide-murder-killings-rate-grew-2019/2795920001/.

79 **mostly Black suspects:** Jared Bennett, "LMPD Report Claims Eight Years Without Police Shootings, Omits Breonna Taylor's Name." Kentucky Center for Investigative Reporting. June 17, 2020. Site: https://kycir.org/2020/06/17/lmpd-report-on-police-shootings-doesnt-name-breonna-taylor-david-mcatee/.

80 **same day Iroquois shuttered:** Janet Patton, "Dining Spots Scramble as Beshear Orders Ky. Bars, Restaurants to Close Dine-In Service." *Lexington Herald-Leader*. March 16, 2020. Site: https://www.kentucky.com/lexgoeat/restaurants/article241225476.html.

80 **two-thirds of restaurant workers:** Mike Pomranz, "Two-Thirds of Restaurant Employees Have Lost Their Jobs Due to Covid-19, National Restaurant Association Says." *Food & Wine*. April 21, 2020. Site: https://www.foodandwine.com/news/national-restaurant-association-unemployment-statistics-coronavirus.

80 **fourth of total job losses:** Jenny G. Zhang, "The Restaurant Industry Lost 5.5 Million Jobs in April." *Eater*. May 8, 2020. Site: https://www.eater.com/2020/5/8/21251960/restaurant-industry-jobs-lost-unemployment-april-coronavirus-pandemic.

81 **he would draw pictures:** Erica Paterson, "Tough and Universal: Nikkia Rhodes Remembers Smoketown Childhood." WPFL News Louisville. September 28, 2018. Site: https://wfpl.org/tough-and-universal-cooking-instructor-nikkia-rhodes-remembers-smoketown-childhood/.

84 **researchers were already warning:** Emma Dorn, Bryan Hancock, Jimmy Sarakatsannis, and Ellen Viruleg, "Covid-19 and Student Learning in the United States: The Hurt Could Last a Lifetime." McKinsey & Company. June 1, 2020. Site: https://www.mckinsey.com/industries/public-and-social-sector/our-insights/covid-19-and-student-learning-in-the-united-states-the-hurt-could-last-a-lifetime.

84 **speeches aired on local radio:** "JCPS Planning Salutes to Class of 2020." Jefferson County Public Schools. May 6 2020. Site: https://jefferson.kyschools.us/departments/communications/monday-memo/jcps-planning-salutes-class-2020.

85 **20 million Americans:** Rakesh Kochnar, "Unemployment Rose Higher in Three Months of Covid-19 Than It Did in Two Years of the Great Depression." *Fact Tank*, Pew Research Center. June 11, 2020. Site: https://www.pewresearch.org/fact-tank/2020/06/11/unemployment-rose-higher-in-three-months-of-covid-19-than-it-did-in-two-years-of-the-great-recession/.

85 **"She looked out":** "Faculty and Staff at Western High School Remember Breonna Taylor as a Student." WDRB Media. October 1, 2020. Site: https://www.wdrb.com/news/faculty-and-staff-at-western-high-school-remember-breonna-taylor-as-a-student/article_b4640c8e-0429-11eb-830f-4be4ceabbcf9.html.

85 **liked babies but not kids:** Christine Pelisek, "Breonna Taylor's Mom Worried ER Tech Daughter Would Get Coronavirus Before Police Killed Her." *People*. June 11, 2020. Site: https://people.com/crime/breonna-taylor-mom-worried-daughter-coronavirus-before -police-shooting/.

86 **two different emergency rooms:** Duvall, "FACT CHECK 2.0."

86 **Her mother worried:** Errin Haines, "Family Seeks Answers in Fatal Police Shooting of Louisville Woman in Her Apartment." *The 19th*. May 11, 2020. Site: https://19thnews .org/2020/05/family-seeks-answers-in-fatal-police-shooting-of-louisville-woman-in-her -apartment/.

86 **Breonna was reportedly unfazed:** Pelisek, "Breonna Taylor's Mom Worried."

86 **ER shifts that week:** Tessa Duvall, "Breonna Taylor Shooting: A Minute-by-Minute Time- line of the Events That Led to Her Death." Louisville *Courier-Journal*. September 23, 2020. Site: https://www.courier-journal.com/story/news/local/breonna-taylor/2020/09/23/minute -by-minute-timeline-breonna-taylor-shooting/3467112001/.

86 **shot as he jogged:** Richard Fausset, "What We Know About the Shooting Death of Ahmaud Arbery." *New York Times*. November 13, 2020. Site: https://www.nytimes.com/article/ahmaud -arbery-shooting-georgia.html.

86 **more than eight minutes:** Evan Hill, Ainara Tiefenthäler, Christiaan Triebert, Drew Jor- dan, Haley Willis, and Robin Stein, "How George Floyd Was Killed in Police Custody." *New York Times*. May 31, 2020. Site: https://www.nytimes.com/2020/05/31/us/george-floyd -investigation.html.

89 **nearly 100,000 on May 25:** Ben Westcott, Brett McKeehan, Zamira Rahim, Mike Hayes, Melissa Macaya, and Meg Wagner, "May 25 Coronavirus News." CNN. Site: https://www .cnn.com/world/live-news/coronavirus-pandemic-05-25-20-intl/index.html.

89 **officials fretted:** Hollie Silverman and Theresa Waldrop, "The Protests Are Raising Fears of Spike in Coronavirus Cases." CNN. June 1, 2020. Site: https://www.cnn.com/2020/06/01/ health/protests-coronavirus-spread-concerns/index.html.

90 **possibly the largest movement:** Larry Buchanan, Quoctrung Bui, and Jugal K. Patel, "Black Lives Matter May Be the Largest Movement in U.S. History." *New York Times*. July 3, 2020. Site: https://www.nytimes.com/interactive/2020/07/03/us/george-floyd-protests-crowd-size .html.

90 **$1 billion to $2 billion:** Jennifer A. Kingson, "Exclusive: $1 Billion-Plus Riot Damage Is Most Expensive in Insurance History." *Axios*. September 16, 2020. Site: https://www.axios .com/riots-cost-property-damage-276c9bcc-a455-4067-b06a-66f9db4cea9c.html.

PART TWO
THE PATIENT: DOWNHILL

94 **shut down its campus:** Michael Nowels, "Coronavirus Live Updates: Covid-19 in the Bay Area, Friday March 20." *Mercury News*. March 20, 2020. Site: https://www.mercurynews .com/2020/03/20/coronavirus-live-updates-covid-19-in-the-bay-area-friday-march-20/.

96 **intubation boxes:** David Turer, Jason Cheng, and Heng Ban, "Intubation Boxes: An Extra Layer of Safety or a False Sense of Security?" *STAT*. May 5, 2020. Site: https://www.statnews .com/2020/05/05/intubation-boxes-extra-layer-safety-or-false-sense-security/.

96 **cause infection:** "Mechanical Ventilation." Cleveland Clinic. November 29, 2019. Site: https://my.clevelandclinic.org/health/articles/15368-mechanical-ventilation.

THE CEO: DOWN TO KOKOMO

106 **designed their own ventilator:** Taylor Hill, "How Engineers at NASA JPL Persevered to Develop a Ventilator." NASA Jet Propulsion Laboratory. May 14, 2020. Site: https://www.jpl .nasa.gov/news/news.php?feature=7661.

107 **aircraft hangar:** Dave Good, interview by the author, November 18, 2020.

108 **Beach Boys had made up:** "City of Firsts Claims to Fame." *Kokomo Tribune.* July 12, 2014. Site: https://www.kokomotribune.com/news/local_news/city-of-firsts-claims-to-fame/article_2bf5e30c -b1fb-5a45-9c11-e1c44fd08ba5.html.

108 **"City of Firsts":** "City of Firsts Claims to Fame." *Kokomo Tribune.*

109 **a *Forbes* list:** "In-Depth: America's Fastest Dying Towns." *Forbes.* December 9, 2008. Site: https://www.forbes.com/2008/12/08/towns-ten-economy-forbeslife-cx_mw_1209dying_ slide.html#506aaa6614f0.

109 **had employed thousands:** Devin Zimmerman, "Ventilator Production Breathing New Life into Kokomo's GM Facility." *Kokomo Perspective.* April 7, 2020. Site: http://kokomoperspective .com/kp/news/ventilator-production-breathing-new-life-into-kokomo-s-gm-facility/ article_8679a8b2-781d-11ea-b756-cfb9e595adab.html.

111 **an emergency base:** "Airport." City of Kokomo, Indiana. Site: https://web.archive.org/ web/20110718201235/http://www.cityofkokomo.org/main.asp?SectionID=3&TM=3362.089.

111 **The darkness was so powerful:** Chris Kiple, interview by the author, March 31, 2021.

111 **100 volunteer employees:** Jamie L. LaReau, "She Thought of Her Mom When She Volunteered to Make Ventilators for GM." *Detroit Free Press.* April 2, 2020. Site: https://www.freep .com/story/money/cars/general-motors/2020/04/02/gm-uaw-ventilators-ventec/5113005002/.

113 **19 machines:** Karyn Zielinski, email to the author, March 20, 2021.

113 **dozens of residents:** Asia Fields and Mary Hudetz, "Coronavirus Spread at the Life Care Center for Weeks, While Response Stalled." *Seattle Times.* March 18, 2020. Site: https://www .seattletimes.com/seattle-news/times-watchdog/coronavirus-spread-in-a-kirkland-nursing -home-for-weeks-while-response-stalled/.

113 **handful of confirmed Covid cases:** Anita Patel and Daniel P. Jernigan, "Initial Public Health Response and Interim Clinical Guidance for the 2019 Novel Coronavirus Outbreak— United States, December 31, 2019–February 4, 2020." *Morbidity and Mortality Weekly Report.* February 7, 2020. Site: https://www.cdc.gov/mmwr/volumes/69/wr/mm6905e1.htm.

113 **while the virus spread:** Bill Whitaker, "Lack of Readiness, Questionable Federal Inspection Helped Fuel First U.S. Covid-19 Outbreak." *60 Minutes.* November 1, 2020. Site: https://www .cbsnews.com/news/covid-19-outbreak-nursing-facility-kirkland-washington-60-minutes -2020-11-01/.

113 **It wasn't until February 29:** Eric Boodman and Helen Branswell, "First Covid-19 Outbreak in a U.S. Nursing Home Raises Concerns." *STAT.* February 29, 2020. Site: https:// www.statnews.com/2020/02/29/new-covid-19-death-raises-concerns-about-virus-spread-in -nursing-homes/.

114 **help that did not come:** Whitaker, "Lack of Readiness."

114 **Twenty-two infections:** Alicia Fabbre and Robert McCoppin, "24 New Cases of Coronavirus at Willowbrook Nursing Home Brings Total to 46, Officials Say. One Resident's Daughter Visits Her Mom Through Window." *Chicago Tribune*, March 19, 2020. Site: https://www .chicagotribune.com/coronavirus/ct-illinois-coronavirus-nursing-home-chateau-20200318 -bny4f6sx4jbsxcsechcqkbuoge-story.html.

114   **no longer share meals:** "22 People at Illinois Nursing Home Test Positive for Virus." FOX 32 Chicago. March 17, 2020. Site: https://www.fox32chicago.com/news/22-people-at-illinois-nursing-home-test-positive-for-coronavirus.

114   **more infection-control rule violations:** Joe Mahr, "Inside Nursing Homes, Containment a Concern." *Chicago Tribune.* March 22, 2020. Site: https://digitaledition.chicagotribune.com/tribune/article_popover.aspx?guid=2197245e-8c38-4724-91c2-fbd2d19144bf.

114   **food safety, and so on:** "Infection Control Deficiencies Were Widespread and Persistent in Nursing Homes Prior to COVID-19 Pandemic." U.S. Government Accountability Office. May 20, 2020. Site: https://www.gao.gov/assets/gao-20-576r.pdf.

115   **touching and breathing on people:** David Hochman, "Four Months That Left 54,000 Dead from Covid in Long-Term Care." AARP. December 3, 2020. Site: https://www.aarp.org/caregiving/health/info-2020/covid-19-nursing-homes-an-american-tragedy.html.

117   **two hours of sleep:** Chris Kiple, interview by the author, November 19, 2020.

118   **local legend:** Tim Turner, "Digging for the Truth Behind Kokomo's Namesake." *Kokomo Perspective.* May 31, 2009; Updated March 9, 2016. Site: http://kokomoperspective.com/news/local_news/digging-for-the-truth-behind-kokomos-namesake/article_19987ffb-8cab-5263-bdf8-fc5cc389ea82.html.

118   **didn't think to prioritize:** Chris Kiple, interview by the author, August 27, 2020.

118   **Outbreaks would become:** Chris Kiple, interview by the author, January 2, 2021.

118   **just about a month:** Jamie L. LaReau, "GM Just Delivered Its First Medical Ventilators: Where They Went." *Detroit Free Press.* April 17, 2020. Site: https://www.freep.com/story/money/cars/general-motors/2020/04/17/gm-ventilators-ventec-coronavirus/5151821002/.

THE VACCINE DEVELOPER: RACING AHEAD

122   **she collapsed:** Catherine Elton, "The Untold Story of Moderna's Race for a Covid-19 Vaccine." *Boston Magazine.* June 4, 2020. Site: https://www.bostonmagazine.com/health/2020/06/04/moderna-coronavirus-vaccine/.

124   **$100 million per quarter:** "Moderna Commits to $500 Million Capital Raise, with More Possible." *MarketWatch.* February 10, 2020. Site: https://www.marketwatch.com/story/moderna-commits-to-500-million-capital-raise-with-more-possible-2020-02-10#:~:text=on%20top%20of%20the%20%24500,stock%20at%20the%20offering%20price.

125   **barely reached the double digits:** Joshua Berlinger, Jenni Marsh, and Amy Woodyatt, "February 11 Coronavirus News." CNN. February 11, 2021. Site: https://www.cnn.com/asia/live-news/coronavirus-outbreak-02-11-20-intl-hnk/index.html.

126   **ineffective in Phase III:** "22 Case Studies Where Phase 2 and Phase 3 Trials Had Divergent Results." U.S. Food and Drug Administration. January 2017. Site: https://www.fda.gov/media/102332/download.

129   **didn't even exist yet:** Hamilton Bennett, interview by the author, March 21, 2021.

129   **hopeful interim results:** "Moderna Announces Positive Interim Phase 1 Data for its mRNA Vaccine (mRNA-1237) Against Novel Coronavirus." Moderna. May 18, 2020. Site: https://investors.modernatx.com/news-releases/news-release-details/moderna-announces-positive-interim-phase-1-data-its-mrna-vaccine.

130   **blew through its cash:** Stephen Hoge, interview by the author, December 23, 2020.

131   **repeat Covid infections:** David Stanway and Kate Kelland, "Explainer: Coronavirus Reappears in Discharged Patients, Raising Questions in Containment Fight." Reuters. February 28, 2020. Site: https://www.reuters.com/article/us-china-health-reinfection-explainer/

explainer-coronavirus-reappears-in-discharged-patients-raising-questions-in-containment
-fight-idUSKCN20M124.

132 **common cold:** William A. Haseltine, "What COVID-19 Reinfection Means for Vaccines." *Scientific American.* September 23, 2020. Site: https://www.scientificamerican.com/article/what-covid-19-reinfection-means-for-vaccines/.

132 **hydroxychloroquine:** Denise M. Hinton, "Re: Request for Emergency Use Authorization for Use of Chloroquine Phosphate or Hydroxychloroquine Sulfate Supplied from the Strategic National Stockpile for Treatment of 2019 Coronavirus Disease." Food and Drug Administration. March 28, 2020. Site: https://www.fda.gov/media/136534/download.

133 **FDA rescinded the authorization:** "Coronavirus (COVID-19) Update: FDA Revokes Emergency Use Authorization for Chloroquine and Hydroxychloroquine." FDA News Release. June 15, 2020. Site: https://www.fda.gov/news-events/press-announcements/coronavirus-covid-19-update-fda-revokes-emergency-use-authorization-chloroquine-and.

133 **raised questions about vaccine safety:** Helen Branswell, "'They Have to Get the Shots': Trump, Once a Vaccine Skeptic, Changes His Tune Amid Measles Outbreaks." *STAT.* April 26, 2019. Site: https://www.statnews.com/2019/04/26/trump-vaccinations-measles/.

THE PARAMEDIC: NYC

135 **the deadliest day:** Patrick J. Kiger, "How 9/11 Became the Deadliest Day in History for U.S. Firefighters." History.com. May 20, 2019. Site: https://www.history.com/news/9-11-world-trade-center-firefighters.

136 **"Chinese Manhattan":** Vera Haller, "Downtown Flushing: Where Asian Cultures Thrive." *New York Times.* October 1, 2014. Site: https://www.nytimes.com/2014/10/05/realestate/downtown-flushing-where-asian-cultures-thrive.html.

136 **CDC wouldn't recommend:** Michael D. Shear and Sheila Kaplan, "A Debate Over Masks Uncovers Deep White House Divisions." *New York Times.* April 3, 2020. Site: https://www.nytimes.com/2020/04/03/us/politics/coronavirus-white-house-face-masks.html.

137 **shut down voluntarily:** Ann Choi and Josefa Velasquez, "Early Precautions Draw a Life-and-Death Divide Between Flushing and Corona." *The City.* May 3, 2020. Site: https://www.thecity.nyc/health/2020/5/3/21247136/early-precautions-draw-a-life-and-death-divide-between-flushing-and-corona.

137 **1,200 deaths:** Noah Higgins-Dunn, "FEMA Is Sending 250 Ambulances, Hundreds of Medical Workers and 85 Refrigerated Trucks to NYC to Fight Coronavirus Outbreak." CNBC. March 31, 2020. Site: https://www.cnbc.com/2020/03/31/coronavirus-fight-fema-is-sending-250-ambulances-medical-workers-and-85-refrigerated-trucks-to-nyc.html.

137 **by Easter:** Annie Karni and Donald G. McNeil, Jr., "Trump Wants U.S. 'Opened Up' by Easter, Despite Health Officials' Warnings." *New York Times.* March 24, 2020. Site: https://www.nytimes.com/2020/03/24/us/politics/trump-coronavirus-easter.html.

137 **250 ambulances:** Higgins-Dunn, "FEMA Is Sending 250 Ambulances."

137 **"Thank each and every one":** Tweet from @FDNY. March 31, 2020. Site: https://twitter.com/FDNY/status/1245027510594801666.

139 **tiger named Nadia:** Joseph Goldstein, "Bronx Zoo Tiger Is Sick with Coronavirus." *New York Times.* April 6, 2020. Site: https://www.nytimes.com/2020/04/06/nyregion/bronx-zoo-tiger-coronavirus.html.

139 **"bus," not a "rig":** Celia Sporer, PhD (paramedic), telephone interview by the author, July 21, 2020.

140 **only 53,000 available:** Alan Feuer and Brian M. Rosenthal, "Coronavirus in N.Y.: 'Astronomical' Surge Leads to Quarantine Warning." *New York Times.* March 24, 2020. Site: https://www.nytimes.com/2020/03/24/nyregion/coronavirus-new-york-apex-andrew-cuomo.html.

142 **"shit-magnet":** Stephen Hall, email to the author, July 7, 2020.

144 **first cardiac arrest:** Colleague of Paul Cary's, telephone interview by the author, September 28, 2020.

THE NURSE: TESTING SHORTAGE

146 **New York's transit workers:** Christina Goldbaum, "41 Transit Workers Dead: Crisis Takes Staggering Toll on Subways." *New York Times.* April 8, 2020. Site: https://www.nytimes.com/2020/04/08/nyregion/coronavirus-nyc-mta-subway.html.

146 **87 percent:** Michelle Gonzalez, interview by the author, August 13, 2020.

146 **faulty tests:** Michael D. Shear, Abby Goodnough, Sheila Kaplan, Sheri Fink, Katie Thomas, and Noah Weiland, "The Lost Month: How a Failure to Test Blinded the U.S. to Covid-19." *New York Times.* March 28, 2020. Site: https://www.nytimes.com/2020/03/28/us/testing-coronavirus-pandemic.html.

146 **restricted who could be tested:** Jessica Wang, Lindsay Huth, and Taylor Umlauf, "How the CDC's Restrictive Testing Guidelines Hid the Coronavirus Epidemic." *Wall Street Journal.* March 22, 2020. Site: https://www.wsj.com/articles/how-the-cdcs-restrictive-testing-guidelines-hid-the-coronavirus-epidemic-11584882001.

149 **South Korea:** Simon Denyer and Min Joo Kim, "South Korea Is Doing 10,000 Coronavirus Tests a Day." *Washington Post.* March 19, 2020. Site: https://www.seattletimes.com/nation-world/south-korea-is-doing-10000-coronavirus-tests-a-day/.

150 **governor had just been bragging:** Andrew Cuomo, Coronavirus Briefing Transcript. April 1, 2020. Site: https://www.rev.com/blog/transcripts/andrew-cuomo-new-york-coronavirus-briefing-transcript-april-1.

153 **James Goodrich:** Wayne Drash, "Neurosurgeon Famous for Separating Conjoined Twins Died of Covid-19. His Real Legacy Was His Humanity." *Washington Post.* April 1, 2020. Site: https://www.washingtonpost.com/lifestyle/2020/04/01/neurosurgeon-who-became-famous-separating-conjoined-twins-died-covid-19-his-real-legacy-is-his-humanity/.

156 **surpassing that of 9/11:** Dana Rubinstein, "New York's Death Toll Surpasses That of 9/11." *Politico New York.* April 3, 2020. Site: https://www.politico.com/states/new-york/albany/story/2020/04/03/new-yorks-coronavirus-death-toll-surpasses-that-of-9-11-1271374.

156 **more than doubling:** Jennifer Millman, "New York Has Most Covid Cases in World, Deaths Top 7k as Curve Starts to Flatten." NBC New York. April 9, 2020. Site: https://www.nbcnewyork.com/news/local/new-york-has-most-covid-19-cases-in-globe-cuomo-warns-of-more-death-even-as-curve-flattens/2366721/.

156 **New York's flags:** Jennifer Millman, "New York Has Most Covid Cases in World."

157 **than any *country*:** "Coronavirus: New York Has More Cases Than Any Country." BBC. April 10, 2020. Site: https://www.bbc.com/news/world-us-canada-52239261.

157 **triple its normal volume:** Jon Hamilton, "New Evidence Suggests Covid-19 Patients on Ventilators Usually Survive." NPR. May 15, 2020. Site: https://wamu.org/story/20/05/15/new-evidence-suggests-covid-19-patients-on-ventilators-usually-survive/.

THE CHEF: MADE WITH LOVE

160 **anguished 911 call:** Darcy Costello and Tessa Duvall, "911 Call from Breonna Taylor Shoot-
     ing: 'Somebody Kicked in the Door and Shot My Girlfriend.'" Louisville *Courier-Journal*.
     May 28, 2020. Site: https://www.courier-journal.com/story/news/local/2020/05/28/breonna
     -taylor-shooting-911-call-details-aftermath-police-raid/5277489002/.

161 **"God Bless the U.S.A.":** Sarah Ladd, "Beshear Hanged in Effigy as Second Amendment
     Supporters Rally at Capitol Before Memorial Day." Louisville *Courier-Journal*. May 24, 2020.
     Site: https://www.courier-journal.com/story/news/politics/2020/05/24/second-amendment
     -supporters-protest-covid-19-restrictions-capitol/5250571002/.

161 **Volunteers for America Kitchen:** Lolis Eric Elie, "Louisville Barbecue Owner Killed in
     Police Shooting Fed a Food Desert." *New York Times*. June 5, 2020. Site: https://www.nytimes
     .com/2020/06/05/dining/unrest-louisville-david-mcatee.html.

161 **McAtee's Rastafarian name:** Elie, "Louisville Barbecue Owner Killed in Police Shooting."

162 **planning to buy the lot:** Kala Kachmar, "Did David McAtee Shoot at Officers Before They
     Killed Him? Why Police, His Family Disagree." Louisville *Courier-Journal*. June 3, 2020.
     Site: https://www.courier-journal.com/story/news/local/2020/06/03/david-mcatee-shooting
     -did-louisville-man-shoot-police-officers/3135804001/; and Kala Kachmar, "Minute by Min-
     ute: What Happened the Night David McAtee Was Shot Dead by National Guard." Lou-
     isville *Courier-Journal*. August 30, 2020. Site: https://www.courier-journal.com/in-depth/
     news/crime/2020/06/18/what-happened-david-mcatee-shooting-in-west-end-louisville
     -kentucky/5333734002/.

162 **weekend hangout spot:** "Family Members Say McAtee Died Trying to Protect Niece."
     WAVE 3 News. June 1, 2020. Site: https://www.knoe.com/content/news/Family-members
     -say-David-McAtee-died-trying-to-protect-his-niece-570934951.html.

162 **raising his arm:** Kachmar, "Minute by Minute."

163 **get a gun:** Kachmar, "Did David McAtee Shoot at Officers Before They Killed Him?"

163 **lay for hours:** Eleanor Klibanoff, Jacob Ryan, and Kate Howard, "After Police Shoot Man in
     West End, Calls for Justice, Body Camera Footage." WFPL. June 1 2020. Site: https://wfpl
     .org/after-police-shoot-man-in-west-end-calls-for-justice-body-camera-footage/.

163 **"Amazing Grace":** Dominique Yates, "'Amazing Grace' Falls upon David McAtee Gather-
     ing Where He Was Killed by Law Enforcement." Louisville *Courier-Journal*. June 1, 2020.
     Site: https://www.courier-journal.com/story/news/local/2020/06/01/david-mcatee-amazing
     -grace-song-stirs-emotions-protest/5311349002/.

163 **three full-service grocery stores:** Billy Kobin and Bailey Loosemore, "Kroger to Reopen
     Louisville Store That Was Looted Near Site of David McAtee's Death." Louisville *Courier-
     Journal*. June 2, 2020. Site: https://www.courier-journal.com/story/news/local/2020/06/02/
     louisville-protests-looting-captured-video-west-end-kroger/5316302002/.

163 **shear 15 years off:** Taylor Weiter, "Metro Council, Fischer Administration Discuss Declar-
     ing Racism a Public Health Crisis." WHAS11 ABC. July 29, 2020. Site: https://www.whas11
     .com/article/news/local/louisville-public-health-crisis-discuss-metro-council/417-9438c22b
     -39e0-40f4-8f7e-b5a226a70f86.

164 **10 worst-hit cities:** Sarah Ehresman, "The Economic Impact of the Coronavirus Pan-
     demic in the Louisville Region." Kentuckiana Works. June 4, 2020. Site: https://www
     .kentuckianaworks.org/news/louisville-economy-covid19.

165 **"I want to help":** Facebook post by Edward Lee, June 9, 2020. Site: https://www.facebook
     .com/permalink.php?story_fbid=10221496570139140&id=1097868933.

166 **well-wishers honked:** Deborah Yetter, "Car Cavalcade Greets Crestwood Mom Recovered from Covid-19 After 43-Day Hospital Stay." Louisville *Courier-Journal.* May 20, 2020. Site: https://www.courier-journal.com/story/news/local/2020/05/20/coronavirus-kentucky-car -parade-greets-mom-recovered-covid-19/5229543002/.

167 **big new donations:** "$1.3 Million Contribution Made to SummerWorks Program." WLKY. June 16, 2020. Site: https://www.wlky.com/article/mayor-gives-update-on-summerworks -program/32879640.

172 **false positives:** "Potential for False Positive Results with Antigen Tests for Rapid Detection of SARS-CoV-2—Letter to Clinical Laboratory Staff and Health Care Providers." U.S. Food and Drug Administration. November 3, 2020. Site: https://www.fda.gov/medical-devices/ letters-health-care-providers/potential-false-positive-results-antigen-tests-rapid-detection -sars-cov-2-letter-clinical-laboratory.

173 **pretty much given up:** Jennifer Steinhauer and Abby Goodnough, "Contact Tracing Is Failing in Many States. Here's Why." *New York Times.* July 31, 2020. Site: https://www.nytimes .com/2020/07/31/health/covid-contact-tracing-tests.html.

PART THREE
THE PATIENT: WAKING UP

178 **running out of sedatives:** Julia Hollingsworth, Adam Renton, Joshua Berlinger, Mike Hayes, and Meg Wagner, "March 31 Coronavirus News." CNN.com. March 31, 2020. Site: https://www.cnn.com/world/live-news/coronavirus-pandemic-03-31-20/index.html.

178 **set a new record:** Jessie Yeung, Brett McKeehan, Amy Woodyatt, Fernando Alfonso III, and Amir Vera, "April 4 Coronavirus News." Updated April 5, 2020. CNN.com. Site: https://www .cnn.com/world/live-news/coronavirus-pandemic-04-04-20/index.html.

178 **more than doubled:** Hollingsworth et al., "March 31 Coronavirus News"; and Yeung et al., "April 4 Coronavirus News."

186 **early data:** Lev Facher, "Is Convalescent Plasma Safe and Effective? We Answer the Major Questions About the Covid-19 Treatment." *STAT.* August 23, 2020. Site: https://www .statnews.com/2020/08/23/is-convalescent-plasma-safe-and-effective/.

186 **convalescent plasma treatment:** Noah Weiland, Sharon LaFraniere, and Sheri Fink, "F.D.A.'s Approval of Blood Plasma Is Now on Hold." *New York Times.* August 19, 2020. Site: https://www.nytimes.com/2020/08/19/us/politics/blood-plasma-covid-19.html.

THE PARAMEDIC: PROCESSION

194 **seat of his pants smoking:** Penny McGlachlin, Dedication at the Cook's County Fire Station in New Brunswick, Maine. July 15, 2020. Site: https://web.archive.org/web/20080526082657/ woodstockfire.net/fireprayer.htm.

THE CEO: THE STOCKPILE

197 **reassured him she'd be fine:** Joe Cipollone, interview by the author, January 6, 2020.

197 **Debby Hollis:** Jamie L. LaReau, "She Thought of Her Mom When She Volunteered to Make Ventilators for GM." *Detroit Free Press.* April 2, 2020. Site: https://www.freep.com/ story/money/cars/general-motors/2020/04/02/gm-uaw-ventilators-ventec/5113005002/.

197 **Reggie had a *Seinfeld* quote:** Michael Todd, interview by the author, December 14, 2020.

198 **Mitsubishi cargo plane:** Rae Yost, "NTSB Releases Preliminary Report on June 7 Fatal Small Plane Crash in Sioux Falls." KELO. July 7, 2020. Site: https://www.keloland.com/keloland-com-original/ntsb-releases-preliminary-report-on-june-7-fatal-small-plane-crash-in-sioux-falls/.

198 **The pandemic delayed an investigation:** Makenzie Huber, "Officials: Man Dies in Plane Crash at Sioux Falls Airport Early Sunday Morning." *Sioux Falls Argus Leader.* June 7, 2020. Site: https://www.argusleader.com/story/news/crime/2020/06/11/sioux-falls-regional-airport-fatal-crash-pilot-name-not-released/5342978002/.

199 **falling behind and catching up:** Chris Brooks, interview by the author, January 6, 2020.

199 **only three got off alive:** John Hamilton, "Ventilators Are No Panacea for Critically Ill Covid-19 Patients." NPR. April 2, 2020. Site: https://www.npr.org/sections/health-shots/2020/04/02/826105278/ventilators-are-no-panacea-for-critically-ill-covid-19-patients.

199 **close to 90 percent:** Ariana Eunjung Cha, "In New York's Hospital System, Many Coronavirus Patients on Ventilators Didn't Make It." *Washington Post.* April 26, 2020. Site: https://www.washingtonpost.com/health/2020/04/22/coronavirus-ventilators-survival/.

200 **top of a mountain:** Jennifer Couzin-Frankel, "The Mystery of the Pandemic's 'Happy Hypoxia.'" *Science.* May 1, 2020. Site: https://science.sciencemag.org/content/368/6490/455.

200 **inflate a balloon:** As noted by Cameron Kyle-Sidell, interview with John Whyte. "Do Covid-19 Vent Protocols Need a Second Look?" *Medscape.* September 10, 2020. Site: https://www.medscape.com/viewarticle/928156#vp_2.

200 **"we win more":** Jon Hamilton, "New Evidence Suggests Covid-19 Patients on Ventilators Usually Survive." NPR. May 15, 2020. Site: https://wamu.org/story/20/05/15/new-evidence-suggests-covid-19-patients-on-ventilators-usually-survive/.

200 **Newly deployed drug therapies:** Lenny Bernstein, "More Covid-19 Patients Are Surviving Ventilators in the ICU." *Washington Post.* July 3, 2020. Site: https://www.seattletimes.com/nation-world/more-covid-19-patients-are-surviving-ventilators-in-the-icu/.

201 **"prevent the vent":** Jamie Bartosch, "UChicago Medicine Doctors See 'Truly Remarkable' Success Using Ventilator Alternatives to Treat Covid-19." *Forefront,* from UChicago Medicine. April 22, 2020. Site: https://www.uchicagomedicine.org/forefront/coronavirus-disease-covid-19/uchicago-medicine-doctors-see-truly-remarkable-success-using-ventilator-alternatives-to-treat-covid19.

201 **reality of a surplus:** Michael Biesecker and Tom Krisher, "After Racing to Become 'King of Ventilators' U.S. Faces Possible Glut." Associated Press. May 10, 2020. Site: https://www.detroitnews.com/story/news/nation/2020/05/10/virus-ventilators-glut-trump/111686054/.

202 **short more than 700,000:** Lindsey Tanner and Linda A. Johnson, "Hospitals Fear Shortage of Ventilators for Virus Patients." Associated Press. March 17, 2020. Site: https://apnews.com/article/8ae013652d8330eea7e5708809b9d877.

202 **more than 94,000:** Fair Siddiqui, "The U.S. Forced Major Manufacturers to Build Ventilators. Now They're Piling Up Unused in a Strategic Reserve." *Washington Post.* August 18, 2020. Site: https://www.washingtonpost.com/business/2020/08/18/ventilators-coronavirus-stockpile/.

202 **canceling orders:** Michael Biesecker, "HHS Canceling Ventilator Contracts, Says Stockpile Is Full." Associated Press, September 1, 2020. Site: https://apnews.com/article/2f697994ea3e53eb966c58106fd96461.

202 **some of the excess:** Kevin Freking and Deb Riechmann, "White House: U.S. Planning to Ship 8,000 Ventilators Abroad." Associated Press. May 8, 2020. Site: https://apnews.com/article/09c0210cdfce9a9d76c60f57ef00d859.

202 **didn't even have a hospital:** Brock Turner, "Rural Hospitals Face Additional Challenges in Fight Against Coronavirus." WFYI Indianapolis. Site: https://www.wfyi.org/news/articles/rural-hospitals-face-additional-challenges-in-fight-against-coronavirus.

203 **approximately 80-fold:** Lisa Stiffler, "How Culture and Leadership Helped Ventilator Maker Ventec Meet Huge Demand in COVID-19 Response." *Geekwire*, November 21, 2020. Site: https://www.geekwire.com/2020/culture-leadership-helped-ventilator-maker-ventec-meet-huge-demand-covid-19-response/.

THE CHEF: KEEP GOING

207 **couldn't pinpoint:** "Potential for False Positive Results with Antigen Tests for Rapid Detection of SARS-CoV-2—Letter to Clinical Laboratory Staff and Health Care Providers." U.S. Food and Drug Administration. November 3, 2020. Site: https://www.fda.gov/medical-devices/letters-health-care-providers/potential-false-positive-results-antigen-tests-rapid-detection-sars-cov-2-letter-clinical-laboratory.

207 **even 40 percent:** Robert H. Shmerling, "Which Test Is Better for COVID-19?" *Harvard Health Publishing*. August 10, 2020. Site: https://www.health.harvard.edu/blog/which-test-is-best-for-covid-19-2020081020734#:~:text=The%20reported%20rate%20of%20false,infection%20the%20test%20is%20performed; and Suzanne Pham, interview by the author, March 26, 2021.

209 **many culprits for Covid spread:** Stephanie Soucheray, "Close Contact, Dining Out Tied to Covid-19 Spread." *CIDRAP News*, via University of Minnesota's Center for Infectious Disease Research and Policy. September 11, 2020. Site: https://www.cidrap.umn.edu/news-perspective/2020/09/close-case-contact-dining-out-tied-covid-19-spread.

209 **more than three weeks:** Dahlia Ghabour, "With Covid-19 Cases on the Rise, Beshear Orders Restaurants, Bars to Close Indoor Service." Louisville *Courier-Journal*, November 18, 2020. Site: https://www.courier-journal.com/story/life/food/2020/11/18/covid-19-beshear-orders-kentucky-restaurants-bars-close-indoor-service/5912916002/.

210 **10,000 restaurants closed:** Aimee Picchi, "10,000 Restaurants Around the U.S. Have Closed Since September." CBS News. December 8, 2020. Site: https://www.cbsnews.com/news/10000-restaurants-closed-since-september-covid-economic-free-fall/.

211 **close to suicide:** Hayes Gardner and Bailey Loosemore, "'He's Irreplaceable': Breonna Taylor Protest Leader, 21, Killed in Shooting." Louisville *Courier-Journal*. November 24, 2020. Site: https://www.courier-journal.com/story/news/local/2020/11/23/louisville-protests-young-leader-travis-nagdy-21-shot-and-killed/6388181002/.

THE NURSE: ORGANIZING

213 **On May 29:** Kathleen Culliton, "Hard Hit NYC Hospital Has First Day Without Coronavirus Death." Patch.com. May 29, 2020. Site: https://patch.com/new-york/new-york-city/montefiore-hospital-celebrates-1st-day-without-coronavirus-death.

213 **"containment zone":** Eric Levenson and Kristina Sgueglia, "New York Creates 'Containment Zone' Around Cluster of Coronavirus Cases in New Rochelle." CNN. March 10, 2020. Site: https://www.cnn.com/2020/03/10/us/new-rochelle-coronavirus/index.html.

214 **drive-through testing centers:** Sarah Maslin Nir, "In Virus Hot Spot, Lining Up and Anxious at Drive-In Test Center." *New York Times*. March 19, 2020. Site: https://www.nytimes.com/2020/03/17/nyregion/new-rochelle-coronavirus-testing.html.

214 **smaller get-togethers:** Sarah Maslin Nir, "One of the First Virus Hot Spots in the U.S. Is Under Siege Again." *New York Times.* December 5, 2020. Site: https://www.nytimes .com/2020/12/05/nyregion/new-rochelle-westchester-coronavirus.html.

214 **Already a nurse:** Taylor Nicole Rogers, "'It's Extraordinarily Painful': U.S. Nurses Strike Over Pandemic Pressures." *Financial Times.* December 9, 2020. Site: https://www.ft.com/ content/b8c7889f-3259-452e-8313-1a2288a3f948.

215 **$10 million a year:** Melissa Klein, "Bronx Hospital Honcho Made $13 Million in Compensation." *New York Post.* February 15, 2020. Site: https://nypost.com/2020/02/15/bronx-hospital -honcho-made-13-million-in-compensation/.

215 **so did the risk:** Linda H. Aiken, PhD, RN, Consuelo Cerón, MSC, BSN, Marta Simonetti, MSN, Eileen T. Lake, PhD, RN, Alejandra Galiano, MPH, RN, Alda Garbarini, RN, Paz Soto, MHA, RN, David Bravo, MHA, RN, and Herbert L. Smith, PhD, "Hospital Nurse Staffing and Patient Outcomes." *Revista Médica Clínica Las Condes.* Vol. 29, No. 3 (May–June 2018), pp. 322–327. Site: https://www.sciencedirect.com/science/article/pii/ S0716864018300609?via%3Dihub.

215 **Covid hospitalizations quadrupled:** Bernadette Hogan and Kate Sheehy, "Gov. Cuomo: NY Hospitals Close to Staffing Shortages as Covid-19 Cases Surge." *New York Post.* November 30, 2020. Site: https://nypost.com/2020/11/30/gov-cuomo-ny-hospitals-close-to-capacity -as-covid-19-cases-surge/.

215 **openly discussing rationing care:** Hannah Knowles and Jacqueline Dupree, "Full Hospitals, Talk of Rationing Care: New Wave of Coronavirus Cases Strains Resources." *Washington Post.* October 25, 2020. Site: https://www.washingtonpost.com/nation/2020/10/25/ coronavirus-cases-hospitalizations-surge/.

220 **told not to drink:** "No Alcohol for Two Months, Russia Tells Coronavirus Vaccine Recipients." *Moscow Times.* December 8, 2020. Site: https://www.themoscowtimes.com/2020/12/08/ no-alcohol-for-2-months-russia-tells-coronavirus-vaccine-recipients-a72280.

THE VACCINE DEVELOPER: EMERGENCY USE

223 **more than 130,000:** Marisa Taylor and Robin Respaut, "Exclusive: Moderna Spars with U.S. Scientists Over COVID-19 Vaccine Trials." Reuters. July 7, 2020. Site: https://www.reuters .com/article/us-health-coronavirus-moderna-exclusive/exclusive-moderna-spars-with-us -scientists-over-covid-19-vaccine-trials-idUSKBN2481EU.

224 **comparing results:** Stephen Hoge, interview by the author, December 23, 2020.

224 **asked to slow down:** Hamilton Bennett, interview by the author, December 13, 2020.

224 **Another 20,000 people:** Mike Stobbe and Nicky Forster, "2nd Virus Surge Hits Plateau, but Few Experts Celebrate." Reuters. July 30, 2020. Site: https://apnews.com/article/virus -outbreak-ap-top-news-health-anthony-fauci-florida-e3081a60a6abf62effa2e6030556ee30.

225 **70 percent:** "This Week in Coronavirus, July 17 to July 23." Kaiser Family Foundation. July 24, 2020. Site: https://www.kff.org/policy-watch/this-week-in-coronavirus-july-17-to-july -23/.

225 **$52 billion:** Sharon LaFraniere, Katie Thomas, Noah Weiland, David Gelles, Sheryl Gay Stolberg, and Denise Grady, "Politics, Science, and the Remarkable Race for a Coronavirus Vaccine." *New York Times.* November 21, 2020. Site: https://www.nytimes.com/2020/11/21/ us/politics/coronavirus-vaccine.html.

225 **$60 million in 2019:** "Moderna Reports Fourth Quarter and Fiscal Year 2020 Financial Results and Provides Business Updates." Moderna Press Release. February 25, 2020. Site:

https://investors.modernatx.com/news-releases/news-release-details/moderna-reports
-fourth-quarter-and-fiscal-year-2020-financial.

226 **Only about 32 percent:** Alec Tyson, Courtney Johnson, and Cary Funk, "U.S. Public Divided Over Whether to Get Covid-19 Vaccine." Pew Research Center. September 17, 2020. Site: https://www.pewresearch.org/science/2020/09/17/u-s-public-now-divided-over -whether-to-get-covid-19-vaccine/.

226 **Associated Press exposed it:** Jean Heller, "Syphilis Victims in Study Went Untreated for 40 Years." Associated Press. July 26, 1972. Site: https://www.nytimes.com/1972/07/26/archives/ syphilis-victims-in-us-study-went-untreated-for-40-years-syphilis.html.

226 **A later study:** Ike Swetlitz, "Mistrust After Tuskegee Experiments May Have Taken Years Off Black Men's Lives." *STAT*. June 16, 2016. Site: https://www.statnews.com/2016/06/16/ mistrust-tuskegee-black-men/.

227 **research on COVID-19:** Editorial, "Henrietta Lacks: Science Must Right a Historical Wrong." *Nature*. September 1, 2020. Site: https://www.nature.com/articles/d41586-020 -02494-z.

227 **By infecting HeLa cells:** Noel Jackson, "Vessels for Collective Progress: The Use of HeLa Cells in COVID-19 Research." *Science in the News Blog*, from Harvard University Graduate School of Arts and Sciences. September 4, 2020. Site: https://sitn.hms.harvard.edu/ flash/2020/vessels-for-collective-progress-the-use-of-hela-cells-in-covid-19-research/.

227 **two French doctors:** "Coronavirus: France Racism Row Over Doctors' Africa Testing Comments." BBC.com. April 3, 2020. Site: https://www.bbc.com/news/world-europe-52151722.

228 **a third to half:** Shannon Mullen O'Keefe, "One in Three Americans Would Not Get Covid-19 Vaccine." Gallup. August 9, 2020. Site: https://news.gallup.com/poll/317018/one-three -americans-not-covid-vaccine.aspx; and Warren Cornwall, "Just 50% of Americans Plan to Get a Covid-19 Vaccine. Here's How to Win Over the Rest." *Science*. June 30, 2020. Site: https://www.sciencemag.org/news/2020/06/just-50-americans-plan-get-covid-19-vaccine -here-s-how-win-over-rest.

228 **bipartisan supermajorities:** Ed Silverman, "Poll: Most Americans Believe the Covid-19 Vaccine Approval Process Is Driven By Politics, Not Science." *STAT*. August 30, 2020. Site: https://www.statnews.com/pharmalot/2020/08/31/most-americans-believe-the-covid-19 -vaccine-approval-process-is-driven-by-politics-not-science/.

228 **Nearly 80 percent:** Tyson et al., "U.S. Public Divided."

228 **cow-like features in children:** Lisa Rosner, "What's in a Name? Or, Will Vaccination Turn Your Children into Cows?" *The History of Vaccines*. March 20, 2012. Site: https://www .historyofvaccines.org/content/blog/what%E2%80%99s-name-or-will-vaccination-turn -your-children-cows.

228 **darning needle:** Jonathan M. Berman, *Anti-vaxxers: How to Challenge a Misinformed Movement*. Cambridge, MA: MIT Press, 2020.

228 **Within six years:** Gary Robbins, "Peter Salk, Whose Father Conquered Polio, Says Coronavirus Fight Is Far from Over." *San Diego Union-Tribune*. May 23, 2020. Site: https://www .detroitnews.com/story/news/nation/2020/05/23/peter-salk-whose-father-conquered-polio -says-coronavirus-fight-far/111857020/.

228 **high-water mark:** Seymour Martin Lipset and William Schneider, "The Decline of Confidence in American Institutions." *Political Science Quarterly*. Vol. 98, No. 3 (Autumn 1983), pp. 379–402. Site: https://www.jstor.org/stable/2150494.

229 **outweighed any risks:** Virginia Villa, "5 Facts About Vaccines in the U.S." Pew Research

Center. March 19, 2020. Site: https://www.pewresearch.org/fact-tank/2019/03/19/5-facts
-about-vaccines-in-the-u-s/.

229   **trusted scientists more:** Lee Rainie, Scott Keeter, and Andrew Perrin, "Trust and Distrust in America." Pew Research Center. July 22, 2019. Site: https://www.pewresearch.org/
politics/2019/07/22/trust-and-distrust-in-america/.

229   **rates had declined:** Niall McCarthy, "The States Where Vaccination Rates Are Falling,"
Forbes. November 18, 2019. Site: https://www.forbes.com/sites/niallmccarthy/2019/11/18/the
-states-where-vaccination-rates-are-falling-infographic/#4154119913fe.

229   **highest number of measles cases:** "Measles Cases and Outbreaks." Centers for Disease
Control and Prevention. Updated August 19, 2020. Site: https://www.cdc.gov/measles/cases
-outbreaks.html.

229   **after the election:** Sharon LaFraniere and Noah Weiland, "White House Blocks New Coronavirus Vaccine Guidelines." *New York Times.* October 5, 2020. Site: https://www.nytimes
.com/2020/10/05/us/politics/coronavirus-vaccine-guidelines.html.

231   **more than 90 percent:** "Pfizer and BioNTech Announce Vaccine Candidate Against Covid-
19 Achieved Success in First Interim Analysis from Phase 3 Study." Pfizer Press Release. November 9, 2020. Site: https://www.pfizer.com/news/press-release/press-release-detail/pfizer
-and-biontech-announce-vaccine-candidate-against.

233   **2,661 Americans:** "U.S. Daily Deaths." The Covid Tracking Project. Accessed December 13,
2020. Site: https://covidtracking.com/data/charts/us-daily-deaths.

233   **May Parsons:** "Landmark Moment as First NHS Patient Receives COVID-19 Vaccination."
National Health Service. December 8, 2020. Site: https://www.england.nhs.uk/2020/12/
landmark-moment-as-first-nhs-patient-receives-covid-19-vaccination/.

234   **Gustave Perna:** "News Conference on Covid-19 Distribution." C-SPAN. December 12,
2020. Site: https://www.c-span.org/video/?507260-1/news-conference-covid-19-vaccine
-distribution.

236   **"Having concluded that":** Denise M. Hinton, letter to Carla Vinals. December 18, 2020. U.S.
Food and Drug Administration. December 18, 2020: https://www.fda.gov/media/144636/
download.

238   **about 12 million doses:** Jared S. Hopkins and Arian Campo-Flores, "Covid-19 Vaccine's
Slow Rollout Could Portend More Problems." *Wall Street Journal.* January 1, 2020. Site:
https://www.wsj.com/articles/covid-19-vaccines-slow-rollout-could-portend-more-problems
-11609525711.

239   **long lines; crashing sign-up sites:** Hopkins and Campo-Flores, "Covid-19 Vaccine's Slow
Rollout."

239   **doses held in reserve:** AJMC Staff, "A Timeline of Covid-19 Developments in 2021." *American Journal of Managed Care.* April 2, 2021. Site: https://www.ajmc.com/view/a-timeline-of
-covid-19-vaccine-developments-in-2021.

THE FUNERAL DIRECTOR: LAST RESPONDER

241   **77,000 people perishing:** Nicole Acevedo, "December Was the Deadliest, Most Infectious Month Since the Start of the Pandemic." NBC News. January 1, 2021. Site: https://
www.nbcnews.com/news/us-news/december-was-deadliest-most-infectious-month-start
-pandemic-n1252645.

241   **nearly 30 million vaccines:** Jessie Yeung, Jenni Marsh, and Eoin McSweeney, "January 31

Coronavirus News." CNN. January 31, 2021. Site: https://www.cnn.com/world/live-news/coronavirus-pandemic-vaccine-updates-01-31-21/h_1193af5dd1d7cb1a2dcb6c41c1a5ab63.

241 **More than 95,000 people:** Eliza Mackintosh, "January Was America's Deadliest Month." CNN. February 1, 2021. Site: https://www.cnn.com/2021/02/01/world/coronavirus-newsletter-02-01-21-intl/index.html.

243 **Both California and Washington:** Andrew Romano, "Flattening the Curve on Coronavirus: What California and Washington Can Teach the World." Yahoo News. April 2, 2020. Site: https://news.yahoo.com/flattening-the-curve-on-coronavirus-what-california-and-washington-can-teach-the-world-130405639.html.

244 **lifted air-quality restrictions:** Rong-Gong Lin II and Luke Money, "California Sees Record-Breaking Covid-19 Deaths, a Lagging Indicator of Winter Surge." *Los Angeles Times.* January 22, 2021. Site: https://www.latimes.com/california/story/2021-01-22/california-sees-record-breaking-covid-19-deaths-a-lagging-indicator-of-winter-surge.

EPILOGUE

248 **monkeys, cats, deer, and mink:** Larry Brilliant, Lisa Danzig, Karen Oppenheimer, Agastya Mondal, Rick Bright, and W. Ian Lipkin, "The Forever Virus." *Foreign Affairs*, July/August 2021. Site: https://www.foreignaffairs.com/articles/united-states/2021-06-08/coronavirus-strategy-forever-virus

250 **Camus winds up:** Albert Camus, *The Plague.* First Vintage International Edition. New York: Vintage Books, 1991, p. 308.

INDEX